CONFESSIONS
OF A
WILD CHAGA HUNTER

by

Barry Glidden

as told to

Margaret Rose Scribner

Special thanks to:

Stephaine Scribner

For her editing skills.

and

B. Luke Scribner

For his assistance with
the many photographs shown
throughout this book.

and

Margaret Rose Scribner

For all her literary input
and patience.

CHAPTERS

This book is dedicated to my wife, Terry,
for putting up with me all these years,
for her devotion, and most
of all, her love. Without her, I'd be half
the man I am today.
I also dedicate this to my nephew, James,
whose love for mushrooms led me down
the golden path to Chaga.

~ ~ ~

I'm especially grateful to Margaret for her
dedication and unwavering research. Most of all
I appreciate her patience with me. She has taken
my words, given to her in black and white, and
turned them into Technicolor.

~ ~ ~

And to my readers, I hope you have
as much enjoyment reading
this book as we did putting it together.
Thank you for joining me in my adventures.

Barry

Chapter *One*

THE DISCOVERY

I came upon the discovery of Chaga quite by accident. Really, *it was* because of an accident. I had recently been contracted by the Appalachian Mountain Club of New England to restore an old hunting-fishing camp that hunkered down along its trail deep in the rugged forests of Northern Maine. The club had acquired this piece of property and funds for its restoration had graciously been granted by the legendary L.L. BEAN Company. My goal, under their auspices, was to bring it back to life, making it habitable for overnight hikers as they trekked their way up to the northern end of the trail, the majestic Mt. Katahdin. The camp sat in a heavily wooded area known as Chairback Gap, with vehicle access only by sloppy makeshift logging roads; dubious routes at best.

During the weeks, I'd been working at Chairback Gap, I'd been bunking with my old buddy, Kevin, at his home on Schoodic Lake in Brownville. My wife Terry, meanwhile, had opted to remain in Florida where, as a successful insurance agent, she generated the funds to keep us financially stable while I breathed the pristine air of the mountains. As always, my staunch companion was my thirteen-year-old Shepherd/Husky mix, Duffy, all of about 100 pounds. He'd been my best friend and buddy through many previous Appalachian adventures. My other staunch companion was my trusty old 1985 Mercedes Benz that operated mostly on vegetable oil (Yes, you read that right; more about that later). Together, we three planned to head up the mountain on the morrow.

I had spent a good deal of my youth in Castine, Maine (home of Maine Maritime Academy), and James, my nephew, lived in Liberty, Maine.

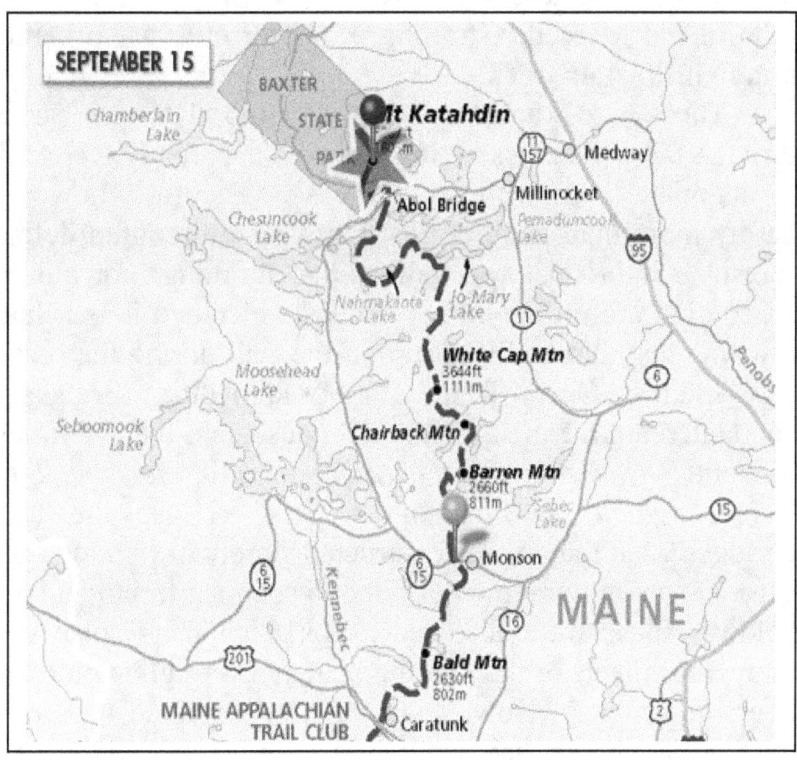

So, needless to say, this rustic northern environment felt like home; very comfortable and safe to me. In addition, my wife and I had worked many seasons at a range of campsites on various sections of the Appalachian Trail. One such campsite received much, albeit dubious, notoriety in Bill Bryson's "A Walk in the Woods."

I got this job through a very good friend of mine; he and I had known each other for years and he would be my boss. I had been bunking at the camp he and his wife, Sue, shared prior to our planned trek up to Chairback Gap. In tandem, we started up the mountain just after 4am, cloaked in the inky blackness of pre-dawn: Duffy and I in my faithful old Mercedes, trailing a quarter mile or so behind him in his pickup truck.

These roads (and I use that term loosely) were carved through the wilderness by loggers who apparently were able to negotiate them with relative ease. They are, however, hardly more than parallel ruts that weave through a defiant forest. A light mist was falling that morning; not quite a drizzle but more than a heavy fog. I welcomed it as it laid-low the dust that had built up on the trail during the recent dry spell. One of the first rudimentary bridges I encountered gave me a moment's pause, and then I blithely thought, *This should be a 'piece of cake' for my light-weight vehicle to navigate across.* (I use the term "bridges", but they were constructed simply of two logs laid across a yawning ravine designed to span the turbulent river below. These were accessed by 2x10 "runners" placed to allow the wheels of the logging behemoths to glide onto and over the bridge.) However, I hadn't considered that, over time, these timbers had acquired a significant coating of oil, and with the addition of the morning's precipitation, had achieved the characteristics of black-ice. I barely had all four wheels on the bridge when I began to slew sideways, then almost immediately, as my tires abruptly encountered the timbers at opposite ends, we went airborne! Our downward plunge stopped abruptly just short of the river and we hung suspended upside-down in a ravine 30-feet below the trail.

9

I'm not what most would call a "religious" man, but I do believe in many things, both things seen and unseen, including some sort of higher power. It just so happened that before I began this venture my auto mechanic (definitely a Godly man) gifted me with a small pocket bible, blessing both me and my car with a prayer. I had tucked the little book into my glove compartment. Now, as I dangled upside-down in my seatbelt, the glove box door popped open and the little bible flew out, landing on the roof, just inches away from my head. When I opened my eyes, it was the first thing I saw. A sign? I'd like to think so.

I released my seatbelt and fell to the roof. I could hear Duffy whining in pain and fear, but it took me a couple of minutes to clear my head enough to assess where I was and locate my pal. He was lodged under the car, with only his head free of the vehicle, writhing in pain. I crawled to him and attempted to pull him free, but in his panic and pain, he grabbed for my hand, delivering a severe laceration just below my thumb. OMG! What to do? The car motor was still running and attempting to turn it off was futile (more about the idiosyncrasies of this model in chapter 4), but this proved to be a saving grace, for the headlights still shown bright and beamed straight up to the bridge we had so recently vacated.

A logging truck rumbled overhead, stopped, and a voice yoo-hooed down to us. The driver heard my answering bellow and began to work his way cautiously down into the ravine. It was obvious that I was whole, in one piece, and functioning, so we turned our attentions to Duffy. Together, we attempted to pull him free. However, our efforts were of little use, and the terrified dog continued to whimper. *"Necessity is the mother of invention,"* and tired old adage or not, it kicked in for us. We fashioned a lever of sorts by jumping together on one of the outstretched doors on the side opposite of Duffy's entrapment; and with our combined weights, were able to pry up the overturned roof, stabilize it, and pull him free from beneath it; free, but bleeding from the rectum. Not a good sign. We fashioned a sling from an old blanket I kept in the car, and together, we hoisted him back up onto the road.

This was around the year 2010, and although cell phones had become a fact of life and I carried one in my pocket, they were completely useless this far into the backwoods. Fortunately, our Good Samaritan had a radio in his truck and was able to call my friend who had already arrived at Chairback Gap. As soon as he got the word, he immediately headed back down the trail, gathered up Duffy and me, and sped us on to the closest veterinarian fifty miles away in Dover Foxcroft. After a thorough examination, the vet pronounced Duffy a "miracle dog": bruised, no broken bones, minimal internal injuries, and with the prediction that "with a little rest" he would be fine. He was. *I was the one with the problem.*

With Duffy safely ensconced at my mother's home in Dover Foxcroft, it was my turn to seek medical attention. A trip to the nearest ER and my hand, and most all of its working parts, was expertly stitched back together. However, the damage it sustained was to toll the end to my summer plans. It would be a season or two before I could expect full use of it again. Fortunately the insurance company at which my wife was employed in Florida not only covered the damages to my car but replaced it with another of like make, model and vintage. It also covered all my subsequent visits to the doctors, plus all my lost wages for the summer.

So now what? This brings me to my nephew James, a guy who treads the paths of Henry David Thoreau. He and his wife live off the grid in a small cabin in rural Maine, and although he earns his living as a contractor, his field of study is Mycology: the study of mushrooms! Well, I've

11

hiked the Appalachian Trail from one end to the other and have foraged in the wilderness for my food a time or two, but James is the expert, and far more knowledgeable than I, of all things that grow unbidden deep in the North Country. It was he who led me down the path to my discovery of chaga! I refer to this summer as my "Year of Discovery". James and I spent hours, days even, hiking the forested paths of Maine's backwoods. He introduced me to all its flora and fauna; most of which I was already familiar with but a number of which I was not. With the expertise that only he could impart, I became acquainted and reacquainted with the world hidden beneath the North Country's forested canopy. Under his tutelage, I grew familiar with the names, both formal and common; the unique characteristics; the history; and of greater importance, the many uses and cures of the polypore.[1]

The many varieties of these, from the more familiarly known, such as the shiitake, to the lesser known, such as the cloud ear fungus and shaggy ink cap, are coveted and even sought after by the Europeans. We in this country have neither educated ourselves nor utilized these gems of nature, while in Europe, the populace craves them. Each fall, gatherers from across the "Pond" descend upon our northern forests to seek out, harvest, and ship tons of these precious fungi back to hoards of eager customers. The favored, and most popular variety, is the matsutake. During this brief harvest-time, my nephew supplements his income very nicely by providing these to the visiting treasure-hunters.   During one of our walks through the woods, my life took an about-face when James pointed to a huge white birch tree with this funny-looking thing attached to it.

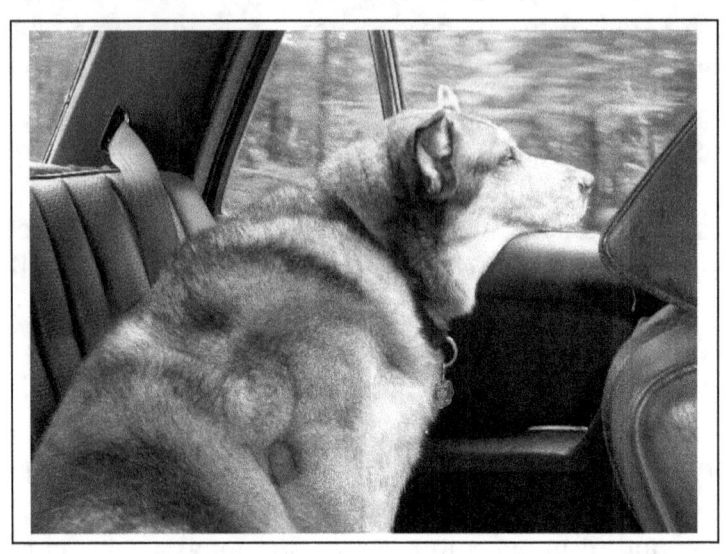

Duffy catching the breezes

[1] *Polypores are a group of fungi that form fruiting bodies with pores or tubes on the underside. Most polypores inhabit tree trunks or branches. Over a thousand polypore species have been described to science, but a large part of the diversity is still unknown even in relatively well-studied temperate areas. Polypores are much more diverse in old natural forests with abundant dead wood than in younger managed forests or plantations. Consequently, a number of species have declined drastically and are under threat of extinction due to logging and deforestation. Polypores are used in traditional medicine, and they are actively studied for their unique shape, some of them being almost humanoid in form. The Chaga have a symbiotic relationship with the birches on which they grow, and often help to heal the trees. If you insert chaga into a dying tree, frequently,*

that birch will recover. If a birch is damaged and splintered at the top, Chaga will fill in and eventually heal the damaged bark. When the wind has caused a tree to lean and rub against another, Chaga can repair the lesions in the bark of both trees. As it grows, this growth feeds on the nutrients and compounds found in the birch tree. Looking at this another way, it predigests the birch's nutrients, concentrating them in a form more readily available to humans. In essence, the chaga serves as a vital chemical factory for substances of great value to our health.

Excerpt from "An Interview with Cass Ingram, MD"
Published by PRICE-POTTENGAR~
~Journal of Health and Healing
~volume 35/number 4 ~ Winter 2011-2012

Chapter *Two*

MY EDUCATION BEGINS

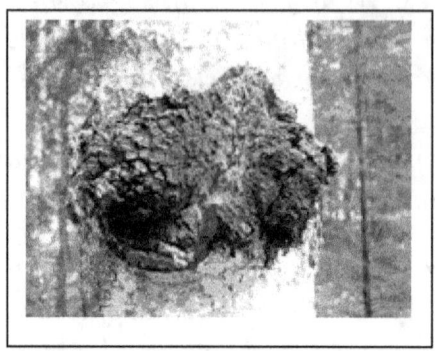

Chaga (*Inonotus obliquus*) is a type of fungus that grows on birch trees in cold regions such as Siberia, Northern Canada, Alaska, and some northern parts of the continental United States. It is of particular importance because it has been found to have a wide range of medicinal properties. Although these fungi are often referred to as "Chaga mushrooms," botanists are not sure if they actually are a true mushroom. Culinary mushrooms are composed of soft plant fiber and are typically umbrella shaped with gills on the underside. In contrast, Chaga are more closely related to woody bracket fungi. In fact, Chaga has recently been reclassified as a member of the Hymenochaetaceae family, which includes a number of other dark, woody botanicals that grow on the bark of trees. On average, Chaga are 8 to 12 inches in diameter, with a rough, bark-like surface, and they may reach a weight of 30 to 35 pounds. Each Chaga takes on a unique shape, some of them being almost humanoid in form.

My discovery of this amazing mushroom/fungus (for the sake of simplicity, I will refer to the Chaga as a mushroom from here on) while at my nephew's home in Liberty, Maine, sent me delving deep into his vast comprehensive library, and I was just astounded by what I learned. The many and varied medicinal qualities of the Chaga mushroom are almost incomprehensible.

"Wanna try it?" James asked. He had a supply of ground-up Chaga at his cabin and offered to brew up a cup of tea. Then, with his urgings, I had my first taste of Chaga tea. The taste was not unpleasant, rather woodsy; a bit like stirring a piece of wood from the campfire into a pot of boiling water. Soon after this initial experience with Chaga tea, I left James's cabin to visit my friends Tom and Debby in Windham, located some distance away in southern Maine. On the drive there, I began to experience a new and pleasant sensation sweeping over and through me; a feeling of being deeply at peace. *There was something very different going on here, within the inner me, and I knew it had to be from the Chaga tea.*

For years I'd suffered with chronic high blood pressure; a condition I believe inherited from my dear mother. So debilitating was it that, often while driving, this malady would necessitate a quick exit off the road to "sit it out," relax, and regroup, before driving further on. Needless to say, *this* trip was entirely different!

When I reached my destination, I couldn't wait to relate my new-found knowledge about this strange and wonderful mushroom to Tom and Debby. Debby immediately went to her computer, googled it, and printed off reams of information; confirming that this amazing thing, this ugly growth on a birch tree, had the ability to change the health and human condition for the better of anyone and everyone who would have access to it. It had been used for centuries by the Europeans and others in the far-northern hemispheres of the globe, with amazing results.

16

At that point I vowed my mission would be to gather, fine-tune, and communicate this knowledge; making it available to the populous of our own country. It was here, right on our own doorstep! Chaga was about to become a very important part of my life.

~ ~ ~ ~ ~ ~

Here I must harken back to my childhood and early teens. From my earliest recollections, my mother wished, planned even, for me to become a doctor. Of course, it was a crushing disappointment for her when this didn't happen. Even more painful for her when, in my mid-teens, I discovered Haight-Ashbury (it *was* the 60's, the "age of enlightenment," after all). Now, with a new clarity, it suddenly occurred to me that, in some perverse twist in my universe, I might just be able to fulfill her heart's desire. If I could get my hands on enough of this phenomenal "cancer of the birch tree,"[1] I could potentially heal countless ills inflicted upon mankind. Thus it was that, for the next seven years, my course of study was to be the Chaga in all its forms: benefits, characteristics, powers and all earthly applications. I vowed to become *A Chaga Hunter*. Their kind are few and far between. It would require months of living in the great outdoors, in good weather and bad, in the snow and in the steaming oppressive heat of summer; though the fall and winter months are the best time for harvesting. Leafless trees make it relatively easy to spot these gems; nevertheless, they can be hunted and harvested year-round.

~ ~ ~ ~ ~ ~

Up until this time, I had worked in a variety of occupations:

17

- Parts Manager for the first Porsche Audi dealership in Maine (decided no more inside work - only jobs in the great outdoors)
- Built and maintained ski trails at Sunday River Ski Area in Bethel, Maine
- Surveyor for the USGS (United States Geological Survey) in the deep woods of Northern Maine
- Worked as a heavy equipment operator
- Perfected my carpentry skills working in all phases of construction and ending as a
- Finished Carpenter
- And the best one of all - the Captain of a scallop dragger!

Now I would become (for the next seven years) a

- Chaga Hunter
  I liked the sound of that.

Along the way I acquired a wife. As kids and young adults, Terry and I had both lived in Dover Foxcroft, Maine, but didn't know each other, although curiously both our dads had played football together at Foxcroft Academy. Subsequently both our families moved away, but after a stint in California, her family returned to Dover, as did mine. There we met, and ultimately, became man and wife. Equally loving the challenges of the great outdoors, we spent many seasons hiking the Appalachian Trail together and managed one of their campsites (I promised you a story about that episode and it will be revealed in chapter 14).

THE PLAN: I would live a very primitive existence in the deep woods of Maine, alone. Aside from the obvious camping gear, I would be including: a Hennessy Hammock, a sleeping bag, my mountain bike for accessing the old logging roads, and a kayak for patrolling the perimeters of Maine's many pristine lakes and rivers.

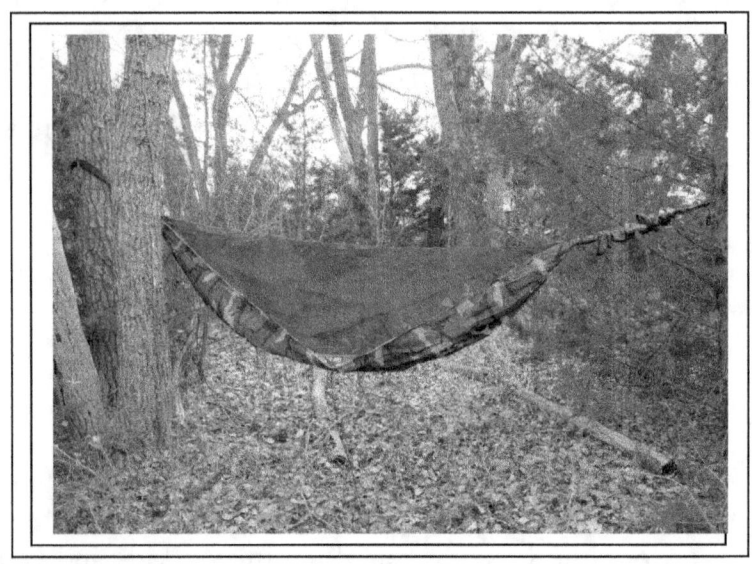

THE HUNT: The Chaga I would seek grows only on a birch tree. It can be a white birch or any other variety of the species, but it must be a birch. The sap from the birch tree contains vital vitamins, minerals, and sugars, mainly glucose and fructose. It is rich in minerals such as potassium, calcium, magnesium, manganese, zinc, phosphorous, iron, sodium, and amino acids. It is also rich in vitamin C and B vitamins like thiamine. The sap from the birch tree is used to make syrup that you can consume directly or use as an ingredient in salad dressings, soups, candies and even wine and beer. The buds of the birch tree contain antibiotic and diuretic properties, while the bark contains digestive, diuretic, and anti-pyretic properties. These are the properties that grow and sustain the Chaga.

THE HARVEST: This process must be done in such a way as to maintain the health and vigor of the tree. Sadly, I've heard of bombastic idiots who have gone into the woods and actually chopped down the tree to obtain the Chaga; heartbreaking and a crime against nature.

To this end, I have developed a lightweight "toolset," ideal for releasing the Chaga from its host. It hangs easily from my belt and consists of a retrofitted roofing hatchet in tandem with a ball-peen hammer with the handle shaved down, so the pair fit together rather efficiently. I use the roofing hatchet like a chisel. The Chaga, when it's ready, tends to "pop off" the tree when you work around it.

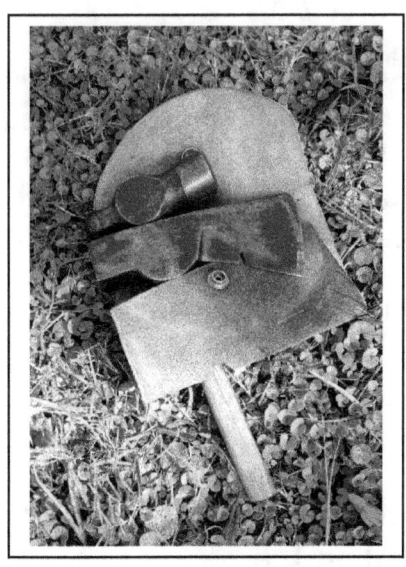

The harvesting of the Chaga is inclined to seem almost mystical; for it lets you know when it's ready to be taken. I recall the summer I spent living with Mike, a professional black bear hunting guide of some repute, when together in his pickup, we traversed the old loggings roads that wove throughout the heavily forested lands between Bangor and Calais, Maine. It was that summer that I became fully aware of the strange and curious power the Chaga appears to possess in conveying when it's ready for harvesting. So often I have walked a path, searching and not finding, when suddenly - there - in the very tree that I had looked at a dozen times before *was a Chaga*, almost saying "take me, I'm ready!" (Not to get too much into the mystical aspects of this mushroom, but as witness to this phenomenon thousands of times, I've come to believe that, not only does the Chaga let the seeker know when it's ready, but it also chooses who it will surrender itself to.)

~ ~ ~ ~ ~ ~

Regarding my long stints of isolation deep in the forests, I'm frequently asked, "Aren't you afraid to be out there all alone? There are bears, and all manner of dangerous critters, living in those woods."

On the contrary, I find it exhilarating, and so, my answer is always not just *"No"* but *"Hell, no!"* I've shared my living space many a time or two with each and every one of those "dangerous" critters, including black bears. Not only have I never been harmed, threatened, or maimed by any of them, but to the contrary, I've experienced a great relationship with them, especially, one bear in particular. (Later, in chapter 8, I'll tweak

21

your imagination with this tale.)

Alexander Solzhenitsyn[1] has a marvelous passage about this very subject in chapter 11 of his book *Cancer Ward* when he speaks of the harvesting of the Chaga. *"He could not imagine any greater joy than to go away into the woods for months on end, to break off this Chaga, crumble it, boil it up on a campfire, drink it and get well like an animal. To walk through the forest for months, to know no other care than to get better! Just as a dog goes to search for some mysterious grass that will save him".*

Chapter *Three*

THE WOW FACTOR

Where Nature, Health & Harmony Come Together

<u>Wild</u> Chaga, (vs. "cultivated" Chaga - more about that later) an unusual name used to refer to a substance found on a very small percentage, (.025% estimated) of Birch trees located in the cold and pristine northern mountainous latitudes of Asia, Europe and North America. Chaga appears like charcoal burnt wood on the side of these very special trees. Even though you would not recognize it as such, by appearance or by touch, it is actually, a mushroom with the scientific name of "inonotus obliquus".

If you are like most, you are *just now* discovering Chaga for the first time. It is presently gaining world wide attention for its unique medicinal and life extending qualities. However, Chaga has been consumed by some remote cultures for thousands of years for its multitudes of medicinal benefits and looked upon with extreme reverence; often referred to as *a gift from the Gods*. Countless studies have been performed on this super food by many of the most prestigious laboratories and research groups from around the world - though very little has been researched in the United States. The information derived from these studies has been made abundantly available for those who wish to seek it. The following information will summarize some of the benefits to human life and wellness.

<u>The Chaga fungus has some of the highest levels of anti-oxidants of any substance known to man.</u>

Scientists have developed the ORAC scale, which is a standard recommended by USDA to measure antioxidant capacity. ORAC stands for "Oxygen Radical Absorbent Capacity". The higher the ORAC score, the more free radicals that certain substance can eliminate. Free radical are like human rust, they are what causes us to age and deteriorate from the inside out!

Chaga has the highest ORAC score ever recorded in any natural food!

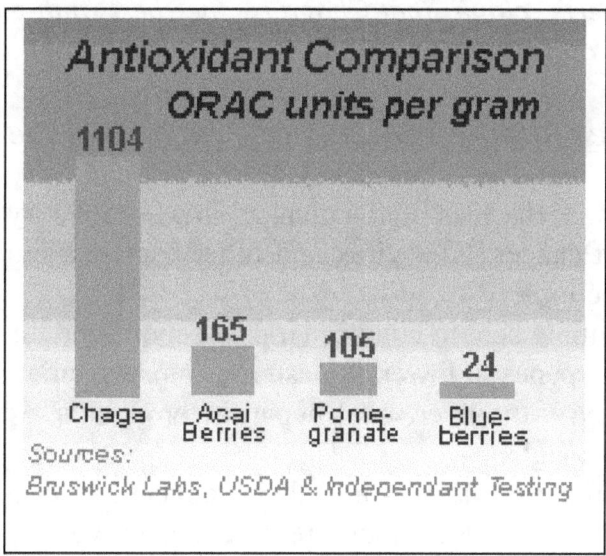

Reams of research have documented the wide range of benefits from the Chaga to include, but not limited to, the following:

- Boosting the immune system
- Treating stomach diseases
- Eliminating intestinal worms
- The treatment of liver and heart ailments

- Eradicating cancers including those of the breast, liver, uterine, and gastric
- Controlling hypertension
- Managing diabetes
- Increasing anti-tumor activity
- Promoting the active compound inotodiol which works against influenza A and B viruses and cancer cells.
- Boosting activity against HIV-1
- Aiding as an anti-inflammatory

Many experts claim that Chaga is the best anti-cancer mushroom of all the considered medicinal mushrooms.

Properties and Ingredients of Chaga include:

- Polysaccharides that enhance the immune system; treat cancer, HIV virus and other bacterial and viral infections.
- Betulinic acid to counter viral infections and tumors.
- Triterpenes to lower cholesterol, improve circulation, detoxify the liver, treat hepatitis, bronchitis, asthma, and coughs.
- Germanium (a free-radical scavenger) to cleanse the blood, normalize blood pressure, and prevent tumors.
- Other nucleosides, phytonutrients, minerals, and amino acids including saponin, magnesium, chromium, iron, kalium, beta-glucan, inotodiol, isoprenoid, and others.

WHEW! What do you do with all that information? The average consumer is bombarded with diagnosis and "fixes" via their television on an unprecedented level daily. The warnings and side-effects of the "cures" are generally far more significant and more dangerous than the original ailment. *Buyer Beware! Buyer Beware!* The consumer has an obligation to educate themselves about the workings of their own bodies, the design of nature and the natural curatives she has provided to us.[1] Our ancient ancestors knew this stuff.

So . . . let's begin. What is an antioxidant, and all those other unpronounceable ingredients critical to our wellbeing? I'll try to keep this as simple as possible.

- Antioxidant: An antioxidant is simply a molecule that prevents another molecule from oxidizing. Since there are many processes in the body which result in oxidation, the intake of antioxidants is essential to counteract some of the negative results of the build-up of too many oxidized molecules in the body.
- Free Radicals: Free radicals are highly reactive molecules that are produced in the body naturally as a byproduct of metabolism (oxidation), or by exposure to toxins in the environment such as tobacco smoke and ultraviolet light.
- Polysaccharide: poly (many) + saccharide (sugar)
- Betulinic acid: is a naturally occurring pentacyclic triterpenoid which has anti-retroviral, anti-malarial, and anti-inflammatory properties, as well as a more recently discovered potential as an anti-cancer agent. It is found in the bark of several species of plants, principally the white birch.
- Triterpenes: Triterpenes are found in all living organisms: plants, animals, humans. Triterpenes are precursors to steroids – in order to produce steroids, the organism, whether plant or animal produces triterpenes. Naturally occurring precursors to steroids and naturally occurring steroids are the plant and animal worlds' way of managing inflammation, safely and naturally.

- <u>Germanium</u>: Though not thought to be an essential element for any living organism some complex organic germanium compounds are being investigated as possible pharmaceuticals. Germanium naturally reacts and forms complexes with oxygen in nature.

- <u>Nucleosides</u>: Nucleotides are the molecular building-blocks of <u>DNA</u> and <u>RNA</u>.

- <u>Phytonutrients</u>: Occurring naturally in plants, some are responsible for color such as the deep purple of blueberries and the smell of garlic. These may have biological significance, for example carotenoids or flavonoids. There may be as many as 4,000 different Phytochemicals.

- <u>Minerals</u>: There is a significant body of evidence that minerals by themselves and in proper balance to one another have important biochemical and nutritional functions. A number of factors have been associated with the occurrence of a deficiency of a mineral in humans: deficiency in the soil; water and plants; mineral imbalances; processing of water or soil; and, inadequate dietary intake.

- <u>Amino acids</u>: The key elements of an amino acid are <u>carbon</u>, <u>hydrogen</u>, <u>oxygen</u>, and <u>nitrogen</u>, though other elements are found in the side-chains of certain amino acids. About 500 amino acids are known and in the form of <u>proteins</u>. Amino acids comprise the second-largest component (water is the largest[2]) of human <u>muscles</u>, <u>cells</u> and other <u>tissues</u>.

[1] *The Cure is in the Forest* by Dr. Cass Ingram

[2]*It is of interest to note that the famous environmentalist, Rachel Carson, recognized the importance of many of the elements noted here which we inherited from our oceanic beginnings. Water is the greatest component in the human body.*

In "The Sea Around Us" she wrote:

". . .Fish, amphibian, and reptile, warm-blooded bird and mammal - each of us carries in our veins a salty stream in which the elements are combined in almost the same proportions as in sea water. This is our inheritance from the day, untold millions of years ago, when a remote ancestor, having progressed from the one-celled to the many celled stage, first developed a circulatory system in which the fluid was merely the water of the sea. In the same way, our lime-hardened skeletons are a heritage from the calcium-rich ocean of Cambrian time. Even the protoplasm that streams within each cell of our bodies has the chemical structure impressed upon living matter when the first simple creatures were brought forth in the ancient sea. . ."

Chapter *Four*

FROM THE FRYER TO THE FUEL TANK

I earlier referred to my 'ol 1985 Mercedes Benz as operating on vegetable oil, alluding also to the idiosyncrasy of its motor not shutting off while suspended upside-down in the ravine. The latter fact probably saved my hide as well as Duffy's for the headlights continued to send an intense beam skyward alerting to our precarious situation down below. I promised to recount the tale of this unique automobile and its distinct characteristics, and, as both the veggie oil and the shut-off switch issues are interconnected, this tale shall relate both.

I'll begin with the unique set of circumstances that catapulted this vehicle into my life. In 2005 my wife and I decided we needed a new vehicle, and coincidently I had just finished reading "From the Fryer to the Fuel Tank" written by Joshua and Kaia Tickell.[1] In this book the couple relates their experience of converting the diesel engine of an old Winnebago camper into one powered by vegetable oil - and driving it clear across the county - gleaning their "fuel" from restaurants along the way. Their book so inspired me that I began the search for an old diesel-powered car of my own. My first consideration was the German Volkswagen truck however I quickly discovered that they were nearly impossible to find. Then a friend suggested a better choice might be an old diesel-run Mercedes Benz. He claimed those old German "war-horses" were nearly indestructible and likened them to a cross between a John Deere Tractor and a Sherman Tank.

He was right!

We immediately began searching the internet for one of those old gems and almost immediately located one on the auction block of eBay! It was offered by a widow from North Carolina, and she promised the proceeds from the sale would benefit the victims of Hurricane Katrina. (A noble cause for a noble cause) It was just what we were looking for - a 240-D ~ 1982 ~ 4 cylinder Mercedes.

And so we started the process. Unfamiliar with the procedure, our friends guided us through the bidding procedures and we wisely set a limit to the amount we were willing to pay.

"It's an ill wind that blows nobody any good". By a bazaar twist of fate it just so happened that on the final day of bidding a hellacious tropical storm, of near hurricane proportions, came raging through Central Florida - wiping out power to many parts of the state. Since the early 80's Terry and I have lived in a solar-power dome dwelling, completely independent of the ravenous utility conglomerates - off the grid - relying primarily on solar energy. Therefore power outages have no affect on our lives. This quirk of nature worked to our benefit on this particular day. The bidding was to end at midnight but as other bidders had no power - and we did - we became the successful final bidder. EBay informed us, via our solar-functioning computer, that we could go to Jacksonville and pick up the car!

Well . . . there was a bit of a brouhaha when we arrived at the Jacksonville dealership. It seems the dealer representing the widow's interest in the eBay auction had concerns regarding another bidder - a collector of vintage cars - who had been heavily involved in the bidding process. He resided in southern Florida and was among the multitude of those who had lost power in the storm. As it came down to the final hour he was unable to bid against us.

Frustrated by his loss he contested our winning bid. Ultimately the dealership sided with us and we were declared the new owners of the old Mercedes!

Previously I had researched several companies that provided the knowledge, and offered the products necessary to convert these vintage babes into cars that would successfully run on used vegetable oil - gleaned from local restaurants. We ultimately settled on *Plant Drive*, a company in Berkley, California. Sometime later I would become their Florida representative and ultimately hire a biker friend of mine, who was a heck-of-a good mechanic, to work with me. Together we converted numerous diesel vehicles throughout the greater Florida area.

The upshot - and proof positive - of this venture's success was proven by my annual trek from Florida to Maine each summer, fueled entirely by used vegetable oil. For a journey of this magnitude I would collect enough containers of oil to fill the trunk, as well as filling the back floorboards. We had several participating restaurants for whom we supplied the containers, into which they would dump the used oil for us to retrieve. The waste food particles would settle to the bottom of these drums, which made the filtering process relatively easy for my wife and me. The restaurateurs were happy to tap into an easy solution to rid themselves of their used oil, and pleased to know it was being recycled for a worthwhile cause. To the delight of one of our local restaurants and supplier one of our Mercedes proudly displayed a sign that read - *"Powered by Clancy's Cantina"*. They loved it! Free advertising!

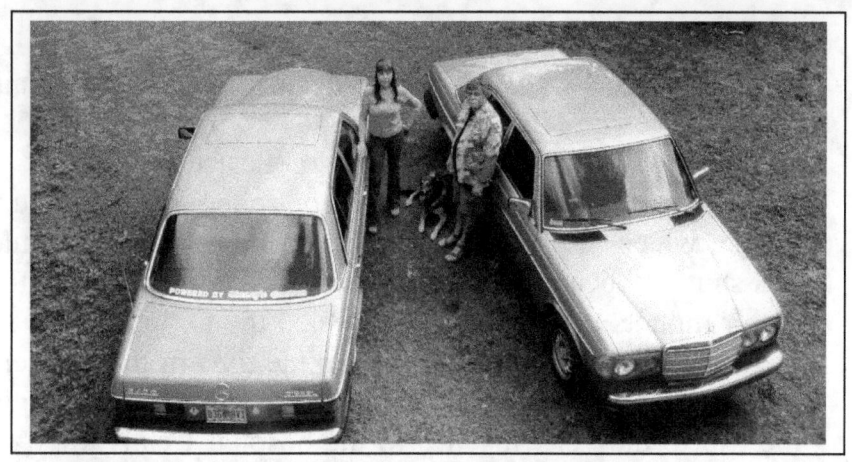

Note Clancy's sign on the back window

On these extended trips north I stopped at all the little "mom and pop" restaurants that dotted the back roads along the routes less traveled. These backcountry businesses had no easy way to rid themselves of this used product so they were more than delighted to pass it on to me. The oil I collected through the summer in this manner provided me with enough fuel for the entire season in the North Country as well as for the return trip back down to Florida.

So successful was this concept - both for the ecology as well as for the economy - that we added a second vehicle - a 300-D Mercedes. We had developed a filtering system that worked quite well in ridding the oil of any remaining solids. However gravity was the first line of defense.

These cars touted on-board special equipment that not only filtered the oil but heated it before it flowed into the engine. This occurred courtesy of the hot coolant. In these vehicles I keep a small booster tank filled with diesel fuel. This perk allowed me to flip a toggle switch to immediately direct the diesel to flow into the engine for each start up - or shut down. Each morning when I turn the key it runs briefly on this diesel until it warms through.

Then I flip the toggle switch and I'm running once again totally on veggie oil!

Now fast-forward to the day of the accident.

These old Mercedes are controlled by a vacuum system which in part regulates the ignition. The car would not shut off because the engine had torn loose from the motor mounts and it had disconnected the vacuum lines, so the shut-off key was useless. From the time of the accident until the time of retrieval many hours elapsed. Specifically the trip to the vet - my trip to the hospital - calls to AAA (they were appalled at the location of this wreck and were unable to secure a towing company to retrieve it) - and finally the successful convincing of a new (young and somewhat 'green') towing service - located about an hour away who agreed to haul it up from the ravine. A total of 36 hours (one and a half days) had elapsed from the time of the accident 'til the time we arrived to haul it up, and the car was still running! When I catapulted off that logging bridge I had a full tank of oil. The tow-guy was able to cut the fuel lines finally bringing the engine to a halt.

I think it's of some interest to note that when the car was recovered from the abyss the only remaining piece of it that was identifiable as having once been a Mercedes was the hood ornament. Nothing else remained of its former self! *And I walked away from that nearly unscathed!*

~ ~ ~ ~ ~ ~

Well now . . . what do you do when you have at your disposal a simple solution that works so splendidly for the economy, and for the environment, and for food purveyors? You take it to the next step! For us it was the creation of a transportation business!

Terry and I now owned two veggie-run Mercedes. What do two entrepreneurial souls do with that? Well, we sat down, thought hard and considered all our options, then came up with a plan to offer a shuttle service! We would offer transportation to folks needing to run errands, attend meetings and appointments and more importantly - to be shuttled to and from the regional airports. We drew up a plan - placed ads in all the local newspapers - and the business was very quickly 'off and running!' The novelty of riding about in a Mercedes 'green' machine - powered by veggie oil -appealed to a great many customers. We were kept quite busy with this undertaking for the next several years, and although most of the shuttling fell to me, as Terry held down a 'real' full time job, I totally enjoyed the experience and the delightful enthusiasm of our customers. ("Wait 'til I tell everybody that I rode to the airport on veggie oil!")

It proved a very cost-effective business as the fuel was free and we could past that savings on to our riders. And although the interest remained strong (even to this day we receive calls and inquiries for this service) after several of years of providing this service we moved on to other business ventures.

~ ~ ~ ~ ~ ~

A testimonial to the wisdom of science in the fuel tank:

Keith Williams, a University of Virginia physics professor, runs his 2005 Volkswagen Jetta on fuel derived from cast-off cooking oil at Hereford College. To Williams' car fuel is a waste. Literally. He and his students run about 20 gallons of waste cooking oil from Runk Dining Hall each week through a centrifuge to filter out particles. They then heat it to burn off any water, rendering the oil clean enough to propel a diesel vehicle. Williams purchased a $1,000 kit to convert his diesel to run on vegetable oil, which included adding a second fuel tank to his car. He needs regular diesel fuel to start the Jetta, since the waste oil is too *viscous when cold; once heated, though, it runs fine in the car.*

~ ~ ~ ~ ~ ~

[1] *"From the Fryer to the Fuel Tank" written by Joshua and Kaia Tickell. "Powered by vegetable oil, the Veggie Van took us 10,000 miles across the United States. The van visited 20 major cities and 25 states where people smelled the clean, french fry-like exhaust. Over 40 million people saw the multicolored Veggie Van drive across their television screens. Thousands attended presentations about the van, and hundreds of thousands more read about the van in their local newspapers." More than half a million people visited the Veggie Van website.*

~ From HOME POWER
#65 June/July 1998

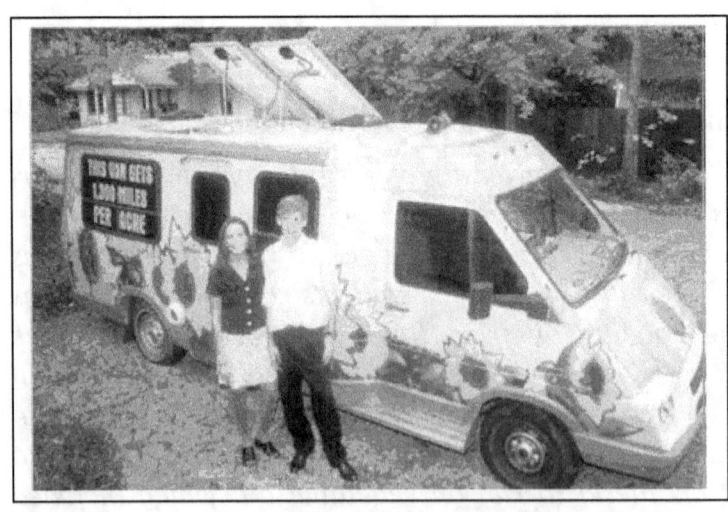

Chapter *Five*

SIFTING THROUGH THE MYSTIC

Oh My Goodness! Reams of information exist out there regarding the Chaga: - the history, the benefits, the pros and cons, the hype, and the blarney. What to believe? In this chapter I'll attempt to demystify the volumes of information that exists on the internet and elsewhere with documented research, and actual case histories put forth by many of the considered "experts" in the study of the Chaga.

Is it FACT or MYTH?

Shrouded in controversy, even the modern day recognized "gurus" of Chaga in this hemisphere: ~ David Wolfe[1] ~ Daniel Vitalis[2] ~ Cass Ingram, MD[3] often don't always agree of many of the facts put forth. For example, there is an ongoing debate regarding the symbiotic relationship between the Chaga and the birch tree. There's controversy regarding how many actual medical/scientific studies have been conducted. In delving into the writings if these men it becomes rather obvious that Daniel Vitalis debunks many of the myths that have come to be accepted by Dr. Ingram and David Wolfe.

Let's start with the **HISTORY:**

The MYTH:

Many websites tout Chaga history dating back as early as 4600 years ago.

36

The FACTS:

According to Daniel Vitalis: "It is very possible that Chaga was known and used during ancient times, but there are no records yet discovered of it."

From Dr. Cass Ingram: "Several hundred years ago (perhaps several millennia), it was determined that Chaga could be consumed as a food. The indigenous Siberians would grind it and put it in stews, soups, and daily beverages."

And from David Wolfe: The Chinese book *Shen Nong Ben Cao Jing* written in 2800 BC names Chaga as a superior medicinal herb. (No original texts still exist)

~ ~ ~ ~ ~ ~

The MYTH:

Chaga was found on the legendary 5300 year-old-Otzi *The Iceman*, the so-named mummified human remains found on September 19th 1991 by two German tourists eroding out of a glacier at an elevation of 10,530 ft in the Italian Alps near the Austrian–Italian border. Researchers from the University of Innsbruck believed he died between 3350-3300 BC. An incredible chain of coincidences allowed the Iceman to remain intact: he was covered by snow shortly after his death and later by ice; the deep gully where the Iceman lay prevented the body from being ground up by the base of the glacier; the body was exposed to damaging sunlight and wind only for a short time in 1991 between the time the mummy thawed and the accidental discovery.

The FACT:

There were two birch fragments around his neck, but no Chaga. One of these was the *piptoporus betulinus,* known to have antibacterial properties, and the other was *fomes fomentarius* used as tinder to start a fire.

~ ~ ~ ~ ~ ~

How the Ancients used it

Several hundred years ago the indigenous Siberians consumed Chaga as a food staple, adding it to their daily consumption. They claimed it boosted physical stamina and prevented the onset of degenerative disease - prolonging life. It is of significance interest to note that in all regions where Chaga was incorporated into a daily diet, there was no evidence of cancer.

The ancients of China, Korea and Eastern Europe considered Chaga a significant medicine and in Russia, Siberia, Japan and parts of northern Canada it is still used as a therapeutic agent. The Ojibwe people of northern Canada regard it as a cure for tumors while in Korea it is used to fight stress and regulate energy. It has been - and still is - used throughout Europe as a cure for psoriasis and eczema and throughout Eastern Europe it's used for preventing bronchitis and other lung diseases.

The Khantys used it - and still do - for general well-being, cleansing (detoxing), and the curing and preventing of diseases in general. They find it particularly effective for liver problems, heart problems, tuberculosis and ridding themselves of parasitic worms. They also used Chaga to make 'soap water'. This was used to wash the genitals of women during menstruation and following childbirth. They found that women (and men) who washed themselves with this never became ill. The Khantys also used the smoke from burning Chaga as a ritual cleaning.

The Chinese book *Shen Nong Ben Cao Jing* (see Wolfe's reference) names Chaga as a superior medicinal herb (though it's technically not an herb). Delving into the writings of Daniel Vitalis, he states that the first verifiable records mention Chaga in the 16th century and stem from Russia. It speaks of Chaga as a treatment for gastric and duodena, ulcers and gastritis. He goes on to say that one of the first users of Chaga were the *Khanty*, an early people inhabiting West Siberia and it's very name *Chaga* was derived from their language. Here I'd like to share an Irish legend quoted in David's Wolf's book: *CHAGA King of the Mushrooms.*

"In old Irish mythology, Tir Nanog is physically located at Mt. Brandon, Ireland, the western-most part of Eurasia, where the Irish Goddess Brigid lives in a sacred grove of twenty birch trees. To those who come to Her, she provides a divine herb (a special mushroom) that grows in her sacred grove of birch trees.

Brigid's divine mushrooms confer healing and immortality on those who eat them by re-activating their Nanog gene. They remain forever young, and are continually regenerated."

David Wolfe also relates that it is unclear when Chaga was first used by Northern Americans. Cherokee descendants claim it was known and used by their ancestors. The Algonquin natives of Appalachia have been using birch bark as medicine for thousands of years and although there is no substantiated evidence of them using the Chaga from the tree it stands to reason that they most probably did.

~ ~ ~ ~ ~ ~

Over the centuries that the Chaga has been utilized and revered by ancient civilizations those early inhabitants derived rather ingenious usages for this gift of the birch tree - above and beyond its expanding medicinal applications:

* It was used as an additive to the diets of newborn piglets. This addition stimulated their growth, and accelerated weight gain, thus producing fatter pigs. It was also effective as a plant growth stimulator and used as an early fertilizer.

* The Chaga can also be used for dyeing textiles and paper. It will yield a yellow or sepia color depending upon what - if any - modifiers are used.

* The Aiun a people from Hokkaido and the Kuro Islands smoked a pipe filled with Chaga, and passed it around among those gathered during religious ceremonials. This ritual was known as *'consuming the smoke'* (Medicinal benefits of the smoke have not been documented)

* The Cree Nation as well as the inhabitants of northern Russia used the Chaga's soft yellow-brown insides as a tinder - or fire-starter. This is still a common practice among woodland survivalists.

* In ancient times the people of Finland created ceremonial drums from Chaga. The process involved coring the sclerotia out from a large Chaga, and then drying it. Once dried its shape resembled a horn, and the prepared animal skin would be pulled over the opening, thus creating a shaman's drum.

On To the issues of today:

The MYTH:

Consuming Chaga will lead to Chagas Disease.

The FACT:

Chagas' disease is a parasitic infection caused by the *Trypanosoma cruzi* parasite. It primarily affects people living in rural parts of Latin America. Recent estimates are that there may be approximately 300,000 persons in the U.S with Chagas' disease who acquired the infection in areas where the disease is relatively common. *There is absolutely NO connection between Chaga and Chagas Disease.*

~ ~ ~ ~ ~ ~

The MYTH:

It's probably unsafe as the FDA (Food and Drug Administration) in this country haven't yet approved its use for treating and preventing diseases.

The FACT:

The United States Food and Drug Administration has classified Chaga as an approved "food - a dietary food supplement." In addition Chaga has been granted GRAS status (Generally Recognized as Safe) from the World Health Organization and it is recognized as a medicinal mushroom by the World Trade Organization. (More in a later chapter about the movement to get approval from the FDA as a medicinal product) Furthermore Chaga has been deemed safe for all ages - from 1 to 101 plus years, and in all stages of life, including pregnancy.

~ ~ ~ ~ ~ ~

The MYTH:

Chaga is yet-another 'natural' offering being fostered upon an unassuming public promoting false hope for cures of seemingly incurable illness. It is probably at best a benign, curious, forest growth that steeps into an interesting tea, but has been hyped by "carnival barkers" as a 'magic' cure-all.

The FACT:

The preceding facts offer historical information and evidence of Chaga's uses and benefits refuting the premise that it's 'just another over-hyped cure all'.

~ ~ ~ ~ ~ ~

Chaga's First Literary Mention in the West

It was Alexander Solzhenitsyn, in his groundbreaking autobiographical novel *The Cancer Ward*, published in the Soviet Union in 1968 and immediately banned in his homeland (he himself was eventually banned from his homeland as well under the brutal regime of Joseph Stalin). His book was later published in English in 1969. In this he details the harvesting of Chaga and the hope it offers the patients who shared his quarters in a dismal cancer ward.

~ ~ ~ ~ ~ ~

The GURUS:

[1] *David "Avocado" Wolfe is considered by peers to be one of the world's leading authorities on nutrition. David is the author of Naked Chocolate, Eating For Beauty and The Sunfood Diet Success System.*

David works, in conjunction with www.rawfood.com, to develop market and distribute some of the world's most wonderful and exotic organic food items. David and www.rawfood.com were the first to bring raw and organic: cacao beans/nibs (raw chocolate), goji berries, Incan berries, cacao butter, cacao powder, powdered encapsulated mangosteen, maca extract and cold-pressed coconut oil into general distribution in North America. Known for extraordinary quality control and ethical production, these products and many others developed by David lead the field.

Since 1995, he has given over 1,000 health lectures and seminars in the United States, Canada, Europe, the South Pacific, Central America and South America. He hosts at least six health, fitness and adventure retreats each year at various retreat centers around the world. David is the founder of the non-profit Fruit Tree Planting Foundation whose goal is to plant 18 billion fruit trees on planet Earth plus the founder of, and leading contributor to, the internet's only Peak Performance and Nutrition online magazine: www.thebestdayever.com.

[2] *Daniel Vitalis is a Leading Health, Nutrition, and Personal Development Strategist as well as a Nature Based Philosopher.*
He teaches that our Invincible Health is a product of

living in alignment with our biological design and our role in the ecosystem. Daniel incorporates the wisdom of indigenous peoples into our modern lives.

His entertaining, motivational and magnetic delivery style has made him an in-demand public speaker in North America and abroad.

Daniel is the creator of FindASpring.com - a resource helping the public find clean, fresh, wild water - free of man made pollutants, wherever they live. He is also a founding member of SurThrival.com, the suppliers of premier, biologically active and fully natural nutritional medicines for regeneration, immunity and healthy endocrine function.

[3] *Dr. Cass Ingram is a nutritional physician who received a B.S. in biology and chemistry from the University of Northern Iowa (1979) and a D.O. from the University of Osteopathic Medicine and Health Sciences in Des Moines, IA (1984). Dr. Ingram has since written over 20 books on natural healing. He has given answers and hope to millions through lectures on thousands of radio/TV shows. His research and writing have led to countless cures and discoveries. Dr. Cass Ingram presents 100's of health tips and insights in his many books on health, nutrition, and disease prevention. Dr. Ingram is one of North America's leading experts on the health benefits and disease fighting properties of wild medicinal spice extracts. A popular media personality, he has appeared on over 5,000 radio and TV shows. He now travels the world promoting perfect health – the natural way.*

Chapter *Six*

IT HAD TO START SOMEWHERE

It kinda started with Charlie. He was a rather 'unique' character. He lived in a camper that he parked somewhere in the vicinity of my Florida home. This was the dome house I mentioned earlier, that I shared with my wife Terry, and it sits in a fairly rural area of central Florida. I don't remember just how Charlie came into our world but he certainly added an interesting 'flavor' to our lives.

Charlie would arrive at our home early in the morning lugging a 12-pack of Budweiser beer and before the day had fully entered into its prime he would have finished off his entire cache of Buds. He loved the stuff. It was nearly all he ever put down his gullet. Consequently we worried about him. His color was dank, his physique deplorable and his overall health bordered on buzzard-fodder.

"Charlie" I said just before he cracked open his last beer of the day, "it's time we did something about your sorry state of health. You'll be dead before your 50th birthday if you keep on like this."

And from this simple observation - out of the blue *with possibly just a few too many Buds* - came the solution - we'd hike the Appalachian Trail together!

Now Charlie had absolutely no experience with hiking, camping or existing at any level without the customary comforts of home and his Budweisers. But it seemed logical to me that fresh air, walking uphill for days on end, and lugging a few pounds of necessities would equate to a return to good health for poor 'ole Charlie. It would also offer me a chance to get reacquainted with the world I loved. He was more than a bit skeptical; in fact he was downright reluctant. However I promised to take care of all the details; camping gear, food, and anything that was needed. All he was required to do was come along as my companion. With substantial trepidation, and a few more Buds, he finally agreed.

~ ~ ~ ~ ~ ~

WHY ME? WHY NOW?

~ My Earliest Forays into the Marvels of Nature ~

When I was still a youngster in junior high, I spent an inordinate amount time in the public library researching and cataloging all of the flora existing throughout the entire State of Maine. The subject fascinated me. I recorded the descriptions, the useful purposes of each plant, whether it was edible or useful for medicinal purposes - simply any and all of the possible functions and valuable applications of each piece I researched. I still have the reference book that I created all these many years later.

In my adult years, I sought out jobs that allowed me to spend time in the great outdoors - frequently in construction. That occupation brought me to Miami, Florida in the 80's working on the high-rise buildings that were beginning to overtake the landscape. During those years Miami was the "wild west" of the East coast - wide open for drugs and all the unsavory elements that follow in its wake. I was then in my early 30's, had a girlfriend - a nurse named Kathy - and we lived the 'high-life' typical of the time and place. Our life style was not a healthy one, and I awoke one morning to the realization that we were in deplorable physical condition and on the road to self-destruction. For me - cigarette smoking had left me barely able to catch my breath. So I proposed that together we quit smoking, start an exercise regime and embark on a healthy lifestyle. We did, and at the end of that winter we were both in so much better shape that we dared to venture out further on our quest for good health. We went to the local Army-Navy Store, purchased a bunch of old back-packing equipment with which we proceeded to walk daily, and set our sights on the goal of returning to Maine to carry on with our healthy lifestyle pursuit.

Though Kathy was a bit reluctant, we did, in fact, return to Maine. Once there, we gathered together additional camping supplies plus tenting equipment, hitched a ride to Cornwall Bridge in Connecticut and as totally green novices, with absolutely no knowledge of wilderness hiking and camping, we set off on a 300-mile journey on the Appalachian Trail. I had brought along several books that chronicled the local plant life and with this knowledge we were able to forage along the way and add to our menu. Surprisingly the trip went rather well though we were ill-equipped - with way too much gear and unnecessary weight. My pack alone probably weighed in at 80 pounds and Kathy's at 60. The back-packers of today would have laughed us off the mountain as their gear is so high-tech, lightweight, and super efficient. We ended up jettisoning a great deal of our stuff early on. (I'm told that with all the gear jettisoned off the trail, a mini-camp store could fully stock its shelves).

That was my first real exposure into long-distant hiking and I rather like it! Eventually Kathy exited my life but the hiking bug remained.

~ ~ ~ ~ ~ ~

Now back to Charlie.

Our plan was to hike the Appalachian Trail from its southern-most entry point - Springer Mountain to the Smoky Mountains, a trip of about 200 miles.

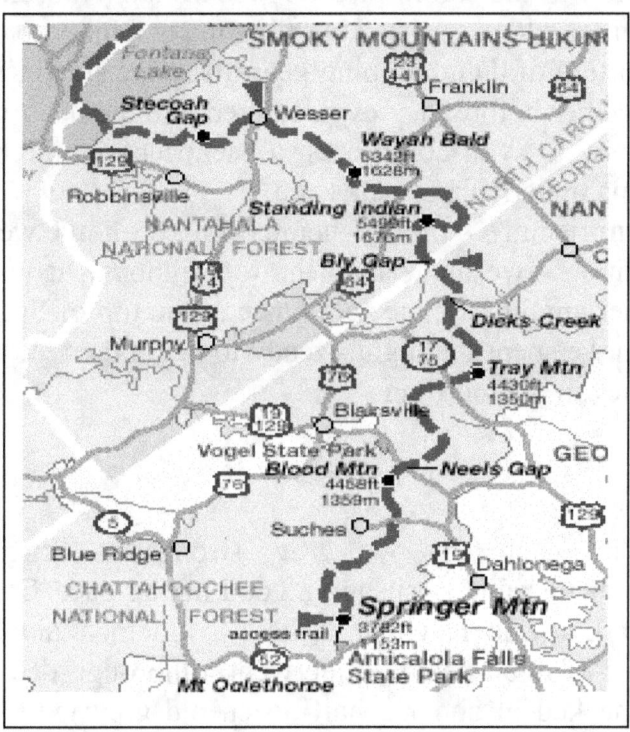

Terry graciously agreed to drive us, and our gear, to Amicalola Falls Camp Ground in Georgia where we were to begin our adventure.

Funny story - while Terry was still with us at the Amicalola Falls Camp Ground, Charlie and I tried out the hammocks for size and comfort. He not only spun around two full revolutions in his initial attempt, but he fell through the side of it tearing open his bug screen! Well he didn't think it was so funny but Terry and I got a good laugh out of it. Later Terry spent hours in front of the campfire sewing up the sidewall of his hammock.

Well, after a good night's sleep at the camp Terry waved goodbye and we started up the access trail bright and early the next morning. This trail is a pretty amazing introduction to the rigors of the Appalachian Trail and the realization of what lay ahead, causing many a hiker to toss a hearty portion of their camping gear off to the sidelines - or quit altogether before they even entered into the heart of the trail! Again . . . you could open a backpacker's warehouse with the paraphernalia tossed aside.

Surprisingly - though neither Charlie nor I were in top condition - we made it to the top, although it took us longer then might be expected. Once at the top of Springer Mountain we spent the night - ready to begin the real leg of our journey in the morning.

~ ~ ~ ~ ~ ~

With each day we grew stronger - fitter and definitely better able to sustain a good hiking pace. Though poor Charlie, who had the farthest to go to attain some semblance of good health, underwent a thorough detoxing. He had packed in about a half-dozen old grey gym shirts and at the end of each day the shirt he was wearing would be soaked in black sweat! This happened day after day until his body had rid itself of all the toxins stored up during Charlie's rapscallion-ous lifestyle! The exercise, the fresh air, the pure foods we were eating, the sweating and the absence of his beloved Budweisers, were all working in tandem to purify his body!

~ ~ ~ ~ ~ ~

It was a time when folks were becoming more health conscious and a company called Fantastic Foods moved to fill that need and began marketing a variety of dehydrated, natural organic soups packaged in small cardboard containers. I would remove the contents - ridding myself of the bulk and weight of the packaging and seal the contents in small baggies. This technique would provide me with a full month's worth of food in a single 1-gallon bag. To this I would mix in a handful of the coveted blue-green algae that grows in Klamath Lake in Southern Oregon. This algae is deemed a "super food" and has even been utilized by NASA for its astronauts. It is considered one of the richest and most nutritious foods on the planet. <u>Charlie would have none of it!</u> In addition to our foodstuffs I would pick rock lichens, little puffball mushrooms, marsh magnolia, Solomon's Seal, and plantain as we walked along the trail so that at day's end these eatable and highly nutritious offerings would be added to our 'soup of the day.' Water is always available along the trail being provided by natural springs and streams. This, however, must be filtered and all hikers include a filter along with their gear just for that purpose.

As preparation for this hike I had purchased a couple of military-style jungle-hammocks. Sleeping in bags on the ground was totally out of the question as Charlie was extremely terrified of snakes. However,
once on the trail we discovered that, under very rainy weather conditions, the hammocks would fill up with rainwater just like a bathtub! Another lesson learned.

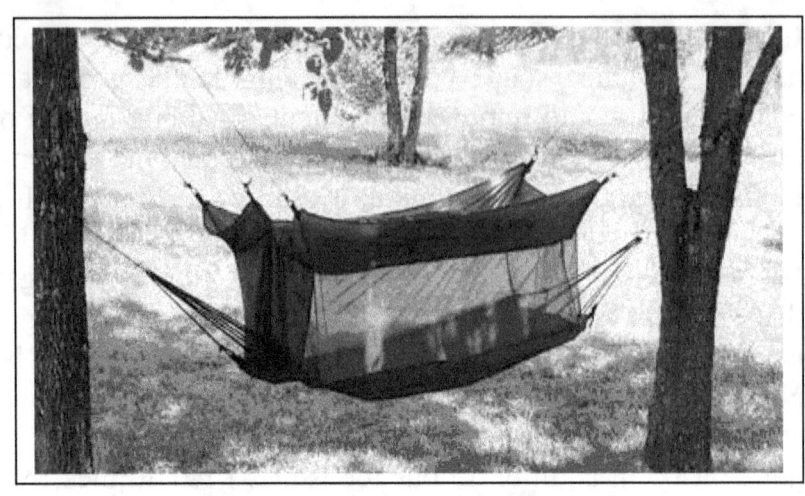

~ A Night of Terror on the Mountain ~

When a big storm comes at you from over these mountain peaks you can see the oncoming monster threatening, crashing, black, rearing its ugly head above you, and aiming right for you. You learn to quickly make camp, hang the hammocks, tie down everything, and hunker down 'til it blows over. On this one particular day we saw such a storm coming toward us. I told Charlie it was time to make camp and hang the hammocks. He didn't agree as we'd gone off the main trail to find a spring and he wanted us to be back on the main trail before the storm descended upon us. His reasoning? In case something bad happened to us we would be found more readily. So, losing precious time, we hiked back to the main trail and began to hang the hammocks. This area had huge oak trees that were crawling with poison ivy vines - huge vines, some as thick as 4 or 5 inches and circling the trees before forging their way up to the tops. By now the lightening was flashing all around us and the thunder was shaking the ground beneath our feet.

Fighting to get the hammocks up and tied to the poison ivy infested trees, while the rain was firing ammunition at us, was an experience I don't wish to repeat. Yet that was only the precursor of the coming storm. We spent the night in hammocks that rocked widely in the furious wind - it was like a scene from Dante's Infernal. The storm was hellacious - evil - with rain pelting our hammocks, entering at will, trickling down the backs of our necks, flooding the berths in which we lay. I truly doubted that we'd survive the night. In the midst of the onslaught the intensity of the storm triggered some bizarre mechanism in Charlie's detoxed brain sending him off on wild bouts of hysterical laughter. These unnerving outbursts continued throughout the entire night, growing wilder and more unsettling with each clap of thunder. I thought he'd gone mad!

Morning finally came. We were alive. Charlie appeared sane again. And so began the task of drying out. We squeezed gallons of water from our clothes, socks, sleeping bags, backpacks and the hammocks - everything. We pulled on relatively dry wool socks and whatever else we had that was reasonably dried out and would hold in and retain our body heat. We hoisted up our packs - now probably weighing an extra 100 pounds with retained water - and stumbled down a forest service road hoping someone would come along. Finally someone did. We got a ride into the nearby town of Suches, GA where services, like dryers, and hot showers awaited us. I watched for signs of poison ivy to appear but it never did. With that we lucked out.

~ ~ ~ ~ ~ ~

Usually when a storm was anticipated, like all seasoned travelers, we'd head for one of the many shelters built along the trail for the convenience of the hikers. These offer a roof over your head and a bunk to sleep on. However, these shelters are also infamous for the cute little livestock they house - mice. Hundreds of them! These little critters have for generations enjoyed the hospitality of the hikers - much to the hikers' dismay. But because of the mouse problem all cabins come equipped with a makeshift arrangement to thwart the pesky little varmints. These are simply cords hung from the ceiling rafters with a tunafish-size can strung midway to prevent the mice from assessing the food sacks hanging beneath. The hikers suspend these food sacks at the cords' end so the little devils can't access them (usually).

Charlie and I had divvied up our gear: he carrying all the foodstuff, and I carrying all the cooking gear, and so it was on this one particular night when we had holed-up at such a cabin. It was our first experience as an overnighters in one of these camps and I strongly suggested to Charlie he take the bag with all the foodstuff from his pack and deposit it in the bucket. Well, good 'ole Charlie rejected this idea. He planned to use his backpack for a pillow and claimed no mouse would touch it while under his head!

Morning came and I jaunted down to a nearby stream to get fresh water for our breakfast oats. (These oats will give you a good ten miles on the trail before the energy runs out) As I turned to head back to the cabin my ears were accosted by the loudest and most colorful cussin' I'd heard in a very long time. It wafted over the woodlands like an evil benediction! It was of course, good 'ole Charlie, and he was furious! The mice had chewed a hole right through his backpack while it rested beneath his head! After calming him down I insisted we empty it and evaluate the damage. The trail mix (gorp) was untouched, as was the dried fruit and nuts, the oatmeal and dehydrated mixes. What those clever little beings *did* eat - *and every last scrape of it* - was the blue-green algae! They knew exactly what would benefit them the most and consumed the most valued food in the whole cache! The mice proved themselves not only

53

wiser than Charlie in diet choices, but had outwitted him in obtaining it!

~ ~ ~ ~ ~ ~

After that debacle we continued on and about 58 miles further up the trail we crossed into North Carolina. Here we left the main trail for a side trip to Rainbow Springs Campground - a very camper-friendly oasis. They boast a grocery store, a shower house (hot showers!), cabins and a bunk house. For economy and comradely most hikers stay in the bunkhouse. Charlie and I spent a few days there recuperating from our varied adventures before we moved on.

This was the infamous bunkhouse in the Bill Bryson book - "A Walk in the Woods" which was later made into a movie starring Robert Redford and Nick Nolte. But there's more to that story which I will relate in a later chapter.

On the next leg of our journey we planned to reach the Nantahala Outdoor Center on the Nantahala River near Bryson City in N.C. This place is famous as a training ground for Olympic athletes in many of the water sports.

~ ~ ~ ~ ~ ~

There is a saying among all hikers "Hike your own Hike". Not everyone has the same expectations, or stamina. Rarely would you join up with a hiking partner that you were totally in sync with - and so it was with Charlie and me. As we continued on week after week our routine morphed into the following routine: I would get up early - make breakfast for the two of us then head on up the trail. After breakfast Charlie would go back to sleep again. He would catch up with me later in the day at the next shelter and we would have supper together. We continued on in this manner for the duration of our hike.

As Charlie and I hiked down the trail to the Nantahala Outdoor Center we came to an intersection of a major highway. As we stood on the shoulder, waiting to cross Charlie began to peer left down the highway - and suddenly his eyes lit up with a look near maniacal. I followed his gaze, and then I saw it too! A Budweiser truck was lumbering toward us!

Charlie stepped out onto the road. He held high his thumb. The truck slowed, and then stopped. Charlie swung open the passenger door, tossed in his backpack, and climbed in after it. The door closed. The truck started forward.

And I never saw Charlie again.

~ ~ ~ ~ ~ ~

This curious excerpt in my life's journey led me one step closer to my discovery of the miraculous Chaga. It further opened my world to the wonders of the great outdoors, the abundance of food sources and beneficial vegetation supplied by nature, and hidden away nearly out of sight - far beyond the realm of the pitiable urban dweller. It reinforced my zeal to live my life in the great outdoors, embracing nature, and becoming one small cog in the pursuit of mankind's health and happiness.

Charlie - I thank you!

Chapter *Seven*

THE LIFE CYCLE OF A CHAGA

WHERE IT COMES FROM:

There are more than one hundred species of medicinal mushrooms that inhibit the growth of various types of tumors, in particular those of the stomach, esophagus and lungs. However, the Chaga rises above the rest and has proven itself the leader of the pack.

Chaga has been referred to as a parasite or 'cancer of the birch'. Some theorize that it is a parasite that enters the wound of a mature birch, grows under its bark until it blisters through and appears in the form of a grotesque black charcoal-like scab. Others theorize it is a type of fungus or mushroom, though botanists are still pondering which to call it. Culinary mushrooms are composed of a soft plant fiber and typically umbrella-shaped, with gills on the underside. Chaga, on the other hand, appears to be more closely related to woody bracket fungi.

Facts that are agreed upon by all who have studied the Chaga are that it grows (almost exclusively) on mature birch trees. These trees are found only in the coldest regions on Earth: Northern Asia, Europe, Siberia, Korea, China, Finland, northern Canada, Alaska, and the far northern regions of the contiguous United States, as well as other arctic regions above the 45th parallel. In the harshest of wintery conditions the Chaga evolves into its highest form - or "superior grade", thriving in temperatures that plunge to a low of - 40 degrees. It also seems to thrive in proximity to wetlands, marshlands, and streams, though they also have been found in trees rooted in crevasses and the rocky crags of hills and mountains.

Some refer to the Chaga as an 'infection', a non-fruiting body, a dense sterile mass of mycelia, with decayed bits of birch tissue incorporated, and typically found on trees ranging from 20 plus years of age to as old as 50 years. Chaga is a polypore - a fungus with pores rather than gills which draws its nutrients from the living tree rather than from the soil.

AMAZING PARASITE:

Chaga was initially classified as a white-rot fungus that grows and lives on the lignins[1] in wood and therefore does not degrade the cellulose of its host - the living birch tree. On the contrary, most agree it enjoys a symbiotic relationship with the birch on which it grows, acting as a healing agent. If inserted into a dying tree the tree frequently experiences total recovery. If the tree becomes damaged or splintered, Chaga will fill in the wounded areas and eventually heal the wound. David Wolfe's experiences led him to believe that the Chaga grows on the tree to protect it - and not erupting onto a tree once it's become injured. He further states that the partnership between the Chaga and the living tree supports the theory that names it an endophytic mushroom, meaning that it can live within another plant symbiotically for part or all of its life without causing apparent disease.

(Chaga has more recently been reclassified as a member of the Hymenochaetaceae[2] family which includes a wide range of dark, woody botanicals that grow on the bark of decaying trees, though not all agree with this)

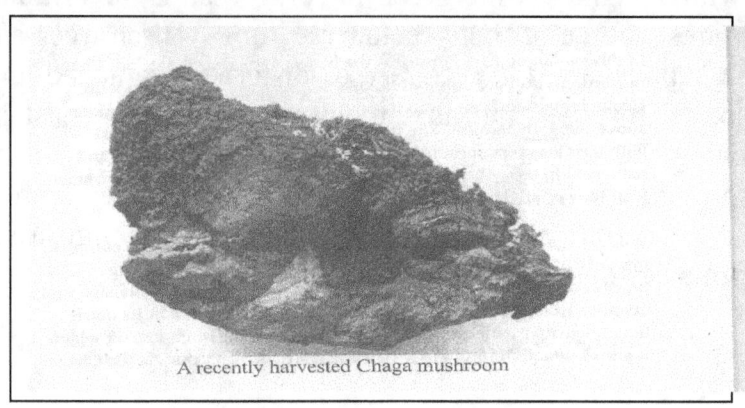

A recently harvested Chaga mushroom

Chaga is not a pretty growth but is a dense blackish mass of irregular shape. It is composed of two visually distinguishable parts: the exterior - black or darkish brown and rich in melanin - the interior has a rusty-brown color, appearing somewhat granular and often mottled with white or cream-colored veins. These are generally classified as the *fruiting body (inside) and sclerotium (outside).* On average, Chaga mushrooms are 8 to 12 inches in diameter and they may reach a weight of 30 to 35 pounds. Each chaga takes on a unique shape, some of them being almost humanoid in form.

A HOST EXTRAORDINAIRE:

The birch by nature is an edible and medicinal gift from the forest. (Remember enjoying a mug of icy cold birch beer soda as a kid? Sadly, the beverage no longer contains the 'real' thing but a flavored substitute.) No other tree on earth can match the vast and varied benefits derived from its bark, buds, sap, wood, and of course, the Chaga. In Russia it is called *The Tree of Life.* The bark, in its own right, is a powerful medicine and a delightful addition to tea, with a slightly wintergreen flavor. Its sap is the original and purest source of the sweetener xylitol[3]. Birch trees aid in the support and the recovery of disturbed, damaged and decimated forests. Like nursemaid sentinels, they assist in enriching the soil, aid in the purifying of the atmosphere, and provide medicinal compounds to the forest's creatures. These are some of the gifts, the qualities, the nurturing elements bestowed upon the Chaga by its host.

THE SEX LIFE OF THE CHAGA

Hummm . . . well there isn't one exactly. At least not in context of what we humans call sex.

The crusty blackened mass commonly called the Chaga "mushroom" is actually a sterile fungal body that precedes the actual spore-forming reproductive cycle of the Chaga. A crusty black conk emerges over several years from inside the tree's cambium (the outer layer of actively-growing tree cells), pushing out and breaking through the bark. It appears to be almost alien-like, and you get the sense that the host tree is in deep trouble. Sometime after the Chaga conk matures, a fragrant spore-producing sheath forms obliquely, drops spores from its many tiny pores, and then quickly disappears. This phallic-shaped manifestation is called a sclerotium. The sclerotium is a compact mass of hardened fungal mycelium containing food reserves. One role of sclerotia is to survive environmental extremes.

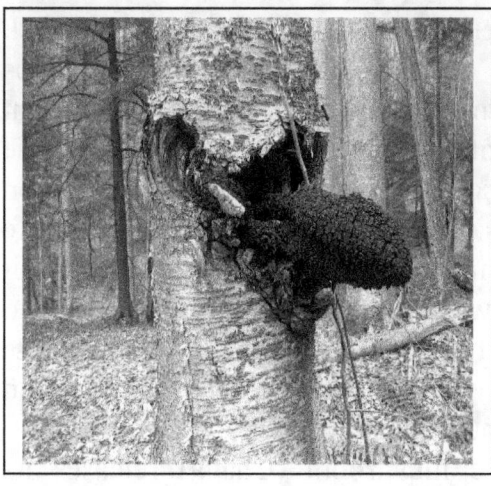

In 1853 Researcher **Louis René Tulasne** proved that the appearance of sclerotia represents a stage in the **life cycle** of some fungi and is important in the reproduction of the Chaga.

There you have it --- the brief, pathetic sex life of the Chaga.

AND WHEN DOES IT BECOME OF AGE?

A Chaga should <u>never</u> be harvested before its time. Never harvest a Chaga smaller than a softball. Leave the smaller ones to grow for a couple of more years. The experts also agree that those growing highest on the tree, as well as those growing in high-altitude areas contain the richest nutrients. "Some of those high-altitude prizes may weigh over 10 pounds. The ideal Chaga fruiting body is over 25 years old." (Quoted from Ron Spinosa[4] in "The Chaga Story.")

~~~~~~

AND THEN THERE'S THAT OTHER THEORY

Did Chaga come from outer space?

According to legend (as noted in David Wolfe's book *"CHAGA King of the Mushroom")* millions or perhaps billions of years ago dormant mushroom spores from distant planets were carried into Earth's atmosphere by cosmic winds and meteors. These spores deposited themselves upon the land and waterways and lay dormant until . . . as life forms developed and moved upon the land . . . a soil evolved that would allow the dormant spores to sprout into mushroom organisms. The final outcome of this process was to establish an ecosystem of multicelled organisms and the eventual developments of lush forest.

When a polypore mushroom (Chaga) releases its spores, they come out like a puff of smoke and levitate upward. They are then borne on winds and carried far distances with their seemingly eventual goal to travel back into space and to fall into the Sun. Their levitative properties seem to assure that once they exit the Earth's atmosphere and enter into the vacuum of space it's relatively easy to begin the long trek toward the Sun. Some may even be hurled into outer planets and eventually out of our solar system. Research has indicated these spores are electron-dense and can survive the vacuum of space. According to researcher Terence McKenna[5] the outer material of these spores appear to be metallic, and lying just beneath are layers of light monoatomic elements, the combination of which shields the genetic material from radiation and imbibes them with the levitative properties that attract them towards the Sun.

The concept that a mushroom can be introduced to Earth from extraterrestrial sources has both a cultural and historic precedent. A meteor disintegrating in outer space - then penetrating Earth's troposphere -discharges enough particulate matter to create the nuclei for cloud formation that ultimately will pour spore-filled rain onto Earth's soil.

Francis Crick, who with James Watson discovered the structure of DNA, theorized that it is mathematically impossible for the Earth's genetic code to have randomly arisen without impute from bacteria arriving from other planets. Then too, British astronomers, Sir Fred Hoyle and Dr. Nalin Wickramasinghe, in researching the nature of galactic dust concluded that it consisted mostly of freeze-dried bacteria.

In the 1930's the new science of aerobiology arose during the early years of aviation, and from this science many spore samples were obtained at altitudes of 3000 meters (9000 feet or 1 3/4 miles). In 1935 the balloon *Explorer II* collected five living spores from an altitude of 36,000 feet (nearly 7 miles). At this elevation, with winds between 40 to 50 miles per hour and temperatures below freezing, it is calculated that the jet stream could carry fungal spores 8,400 miles in one week.

There has been a significant amount of research done by credible researchers who believe their findings validate this "from out of space" theory. For more information read the above mentioned book by Wolfe. He's a believer.

[1] *Brown matter that forms the secondary wall beneath the cellulose wall of the bark of the tree.*

[2] *The Hymenochaetaceae are a family of fungi in the order Hymenochaetales. The family contains several species that are implicated in many diseases of broad-leaved and coniferous trees, causing heart rot, canker and root diseases, and also disease of grapevines.*

[3] *Xylitol looks tastes and feels like sugar but is a sugar alcohol. It is known that sugar feeds infections and cancer*

therefore it is imperative to avoid all sugar and use instead completely monglycemic - and natural - stevia and xylitol.

[4] Ron Spinosa: president@minnesotamushrooms.org
Author of "The Chaga Story"

[5]Terrance McKenna: *An American ethnobotanist, mystic, psychonaut, lecturer, author, and an advocate for the responsible use of naturally occurring psychedelic plants*

Chapter *Eight*

MY ENCOUNTER

There's a Cherokee legend that tells of a Cherokee clan who called themselves the Ani Tsa'gu hi. Their tale is of an unusual quest for their entire tribal clan. It is told that a young boy of the clan kept disappearing into the forest only to return to the village a little hairier each time. The elders of the tribe ask the boy what was going on, the youngster acknowledge that he had been spending time with the bears of the forest sharing their foods and ways. He told the elders the bears had plenty of food and that the rest of the tribe could join him rather than go hungry, but first they would have to fast in order to prepare for the transformation.

Informing the other tribal clans, this Ani Tsa'gu hi clan chose to follow the boy and leave the human world of struggle and hunger behind, and live forever with the Black Bears in their abundant forest.

Upon their departure from the known world of Cherokee towns and villages, the Ani Tsa'gu hi, informed all the other Cherokee clans of their departure. "We are going where there is much food. Do not fear us or attempt to kill us, for we will be ever alive. "

It's not hard to imagine that there are some Cherokee living in the mountains today, who think descendants of the Ani Tsa'gu hi clan might still be living in the mountain forest as Black Bears. There are also tales of how humans might be the descendents of Black Bears losing their fur and changing their ways.

The following story is true. I had smoked nothing, drank nothing nor ingested anything that would in any way account for the experience I will relate here.

~ ~ ~ ~ ~ ~

It was during my trek over the Appalachian Trail with 'good 'ole Charlie'. We were in North Carolina and had been on the trail for about three weeks. As was our daily routine I had risen early - prepared a bracing breakfast of energy-inducing oats, and Charlie, smelling the perking coffee had rallied, and wordlessly we shared our morning meal. Following this I washed up, cleaned up around the campsite, hitched up my backpack, and headed out on the trail for the day.

Charlie went back to bed.

This practice worked well for us. Charlie would catch up with me later in the day, at the next shelter, and we'd share the evening meal together.

On the day I will recount here, I was hiking a side trail (*these are indicated with a blue blaze marker rather than the typical white blaze which indicates the main trail*) and as was the norm Charlie was laggin' somewhere far behind me. This trail would take me to the next shelter where we planned to spend the night. At a small fork along this trail I noticed a curious campsite, not at all the typical kind a seasoned hiker would set up. Sitting aside this simple, rustic lean-to affair was a rather grizzly old man. As I passed by I greeted him and offered him a hot cup of tea or coffee if he would like to join me further down the trail, where I planned my next stopover.

He said "Sure."

So I was not surprised when a short time later he appeared at my campsite, and while the water heated we began to exchange pleasantries. He seemed rather interesting and very knowledgeable about the area, and all the flora and fauna that abided in these woods. The old guy was considerably unkempt, with shaggy black hair and beard and clothes that had been around a very long time. His eyes appeared quite deep-set and rather dark - nearly black - except when the lights of the fire reflected off them shooting shards of red and yellowish sparks into the night that gleamed oddly in the approaching pale of the evening. As he talked, I had the feeling he'd been hiking these mountains for an extraordinarily long time, but when I asked him just how long, his answer was simply a curt gruff reply: "A very long time."

Soon the subject of black bears came up. This area is known as a black bear sanctuary and there are many of these animals that make their home in these woods. Once the conversion turned to these creatures he would talk of nothing else. He rambled on - with an inordinate intensity - about how little mankind knew about these bears, and he began to grow agitated as he lamented further about the need for mankind to make an effort to understand these black bears, and learn their ways. So obsessed and vocal was he on this subject that I began to feel uneasy. I was beginning to believe he was a bit 'off' - and I was wishing him gone. As luck would have it just about the time I was beginning to be concerned about being alone with this strange guy in this remote setting, good 'ole Charlie arrived. I'd never been so happy to see him! With Charlie's arrival the old guy excused himself and left.

The next morning - as was my routine - I got up early, made coffee and breakfast and began my hike back up to the main trail. Then the oddest thing - when I reached the spot where the old guy had been camped the night before there was absolutely no sign of anyone ever having been there. No indication that a camp been there! Not a bent blade of grass - not a stick disturbed - nothing! So pristine was this spot that I began to question my own sanity. Had there *really* been an old man camped here last night?

I put my questions and concerns behind me as I picked up the pace and headed north on the main trail. I was entering into a particular lovely area that is rife with mammoth rhododendrons plants. These incredible works of nature grow so profusely in these mountains and so gigantic that they form overhead canopies with tunnels beneath, large enough for a small car to pass through. During their season of bloom, words cannot adequately describe their glorious assault to the senses. My morning hike would take me right through one of the magnificent behemoths.

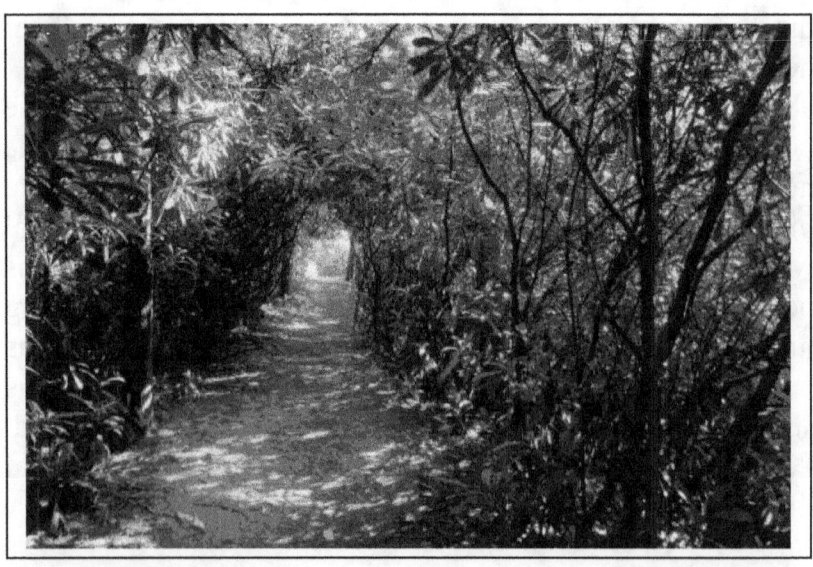

As I entered the tunnel it began to grow dark - so dense was the foliage, and this particular tunnel was quite long - probably 300 to 400 feet from entrance to exit. As the darkness engulfed me my attention was riveted to the light at the end. Curiously I thought I saw something dark move cross the opening, but then it disappeared. Of course I thought immediately of bears as they are so prevalent here and I felt for the 'bear whistle' that hung around my neck. And then again, I saw something big and black move across the tunnel's end. This time I was sure it was indeed a black bear, walking on all fours. I slowed my pace - stopping every few steps and listening, but I saw nothing more, nor did my ears pick up any warning sounds. So I continued on.

Just as I stepped out into the sunlight the biggest black bear I had ever encountered, confronted me. He immediately reared up on hind legs, with front paws stretched high above me on either side and his head looming a full foot above mine. I was terrified - totally petrified! I truly believed this was my end, and Charlie would find my mangled remains hours from now. Then the bear looked down on me - full in the face - and I saw his eyes. *Those eyes were the eyes of the old man I had shared coffee with the night before! Dark- blackish - deep set- with shards of red and yellow lights shooting out from the reflected sunlight!*

I figured I'd lost my mind and probably my life, but just as my fear reached heights heretofore unknown to mankind, the bear dropped down on all fours, turned, and went crashing down the mountainside, sounding much like a plummeting freight train.

> Each shelter offers a log book for hikers to record events they've experienced along the trail, as well as leaving a memo for friends coming along behind them. I had previously noted several references to a "bear-man" many a hiker had encountered along the trail. I hadn't thought much about this anecdote - thinking it was probably woven from the fabric of too much fresh air - over exertion - and maybe just a bit of cannabis - that is . . . until this moment. Holy Cow! Had I encountered the infamous "Bear-man" last night? Did he *really* exist?

During all the ensuing years that I was to trek these hallowed trails, and linger at the many renowned campsites of the Appalachian Trail, we were never to cross paths again.

This story is true. I had smoked nothing, drank nothing nor ingested anything that would in any way account for the experience I've related here.

> *I can't help but relate a joke I heard many years ago. . .*
>
> *In some parts of the country, hikers are encouraged to carry pepper spray and a whistle in case of bears. And do you know how to tell if you're in black bear country or grizzly bear country?*
>
> *Look at the droppings;*
>
> *Black bear droppings will have parts of berries and twigs in it.*
>
> *Grizzly bear droppings will smell like pepper spray and have broken whistles in it.*

Chapter *Nine*

Here's the Skinny

The Chaga's nickname is the "Mushroom of Immortality"

So let's talk about specifics. Exactly what do the 'experts' have to say about just what Chaga can, and will, do for you? What will it cure? What will it prevent? What will it make stronger?

~ ~ ~ ~ ~ ~

We are bombarded daily with advertisements for medications - those both doctor-prescribed and those purchased 'over the counter'. Let's begin with noting many (but not nearly all) of the side effects of these countless medicines:

* Possibly loss of sense of smell and/or taste
* Possible ringing in the ears
* Possible blurred Vision
* Possibly may cause hallucinations
* Possible night terrors/nightmares
* Possible sleepwalking
* Possible heart palpitations
* Hives
* Swollen tongue
* Constipation
* Possible amnesia/short-term memory loss
* Recently revealed connection between acid
  reflex meds and early onset of Alzheimers
And possibly the nastiest one of all:
* Possible uncontrollable bowel movements

70

(The user is cautioned to wear dark-colored clothing)
And definitely the most frightening one of all:
    * Possible suicidal thoughts and actions

And now for the possible side effects from wild Chaga? (As quoted from Dr. Ron McDow's book
"Wild CHAGA")[1]

"The only known side effect of wild Chaga is excellent health."

~ ~ ~ ~ ~ ~

    Chaga is rich in natural antioxidants and anti-inflammatory phenols, containing the compounds betulin and betulinic acid - which are derived directly from its host birch tree. Both betulin and betulinic acid have demonstrated anti-tumor effects, which explain why Chaga is considered as an anti-cancer agent. Additionally, some science shows that betulin can play a beneficial role in controlling metabolic disorders, such as obesity and metabolic syndrome. A group of compounds also found in Chaga, called lanostanoids, appear to play significant anti-cancer roles.

    The exact anti-cancer activity of Chaga is not completely understood. Some compounds in the fungus boost immune activity, some specifically prevent cancer cells from replicating, and others cause premature cancer cell death. This argues for the utilization of a whole Chaga extract, rather than isolating a single compound. In Chaga, many agents appear to be active against cancer (per *Chris Kilham*.) [2]

The Food and Drug Administration has classified Chaga as a "dietary supplement" --- NOT A MEDICATION --- a "dietary supplement" is defined as a product intended for ingestion that adds nutritional value to one's diet. A "dietary ingredient" may be one, or any combination, of the following substances: a vitamin, a mineral, an herb or other botanical.

Having made that clear, the following disorders (diseases) of the human condition have been researched by those who believe in the curative powers of the Chaga. Many European and Asian countries have conducted extensive scientific studies confirming the benefits for those who suffer from the following maladies. We will discuss only the attributes of WILD CHAGA (that which is harvested in the wild from birch trees above the 45th parallel.) Synthetic, or cultivated Chaga, will be discussed in a later chapter.

WILD CHAGA
Wild Chaga is known to contain the following nutrients and natural medicines:

Water-soluble polysaccharides
Alcohol-soluble polysaccharides
Protein-bound polysaccharides
Beta-Glucans polysaccharide
Lanostane triterpenoids
Betulin and betulinic acid
Ergosterol peroxides
Lanosterols (trametenolic acid)
Superoxide dismutase (SOD)
Inotodiol
Saponin
Melanin

Trace minerals:

antimony	barium
bismuth	boron
germanium	copper
manganese	strontium
zinc	

Major minerals:

calcium	cesium
iron	magnesium
phosphorus	potassium
rubidium	silicon

Vitamins: B2, B3, D2, K1

Dietary fiber

Amino acids

One of the most important, and prevalent, component found in Chaga is the Beta-Glucans. These normalize the immune system. An overactive immune system can be the underlining cause of a bevy of woes: allergies, lupus, and psoriasis, to name a few. Our immune system is at the core of our health, and is under siege constantly. Stress, the side effects of medications, and the maladies of ageing are but a few of the issues that contribute to mineral deficiencies[3] here in America.

There have been over 1600 research papers reporting on Beta Glucan. Among them are: Harvard Medical School, the National Cancer Institute, and the Dept. of Agriculture. The match between Beta-Glucan and the immune system has been likened to a key-and-lock arrangement. The Beta-Glucans are the 'keys' and the 'locks' are the receptors of our immune system. Chaga is a 'Living Pharmacy' and a 'Living Ecosystem'.

Chaga not only balances the immune system but optimizes the natural resistance to diseases and infections. The following is a list of those conditions that respond favorably to Beta-Glucans.

Abdominal adhesions	abdominal sepsis
Acute renal failure	Allergies
Anthrax poisoning	autoimmune disorders
Cancer	Carcinoma
Chromoblastomycois	Chronic fatigue syndrome
Cold sores	colorectal surgery
Coronary artery disease	Dermatitis
Diabetes	E. coli infections
Exercise stress	Fibromyalgia
Free-radical damage	fungal disease
Heart disease	Hepatitis
Herpes	High LDL cholesterol
Leprosy	Leucopenia
Peritonitis	
Psoriasis	Leukemia
Pneumonia	Lipid metabolism disorder
Rabies	Radiation damage
Liver damage	Rheumatoid arthritis
Sarcoma	Low platelet production
Lung damage	Skin regeneration
Lupus	Spinal cord injury
Malaria	Staph infection
Melanoma	Stem-cell transplant
Microbial infection	Trauma recovery
Multiple sclerosis	Tuberculosis
Mycotoxins	Ulcers
Oxidation damage	Wound healing
Parasites	Viral infections

SO WHAT DOES ALL THIS MEAN FOR US?

All of these facts and fancy words gleaned from years of research, done around the globe through competent scientific study, mean nothing to the general public if one simply does not understand the impact these properties can have on their own wellbeing.

Listed here are samplings of some of the more common malfunctions that the human body is prone to, which have been shown to be alleviated, or totally eradicated, by the addition of Chaga into the sufferer's <u>daily</u> diets.

The antioxidant power of the Chaga can be compared to *'an anti-rust treatment and a polishing for the entire body and its inner organs'*.

Can you throw away all your medications?
Well . . . maybe . . .

CHAGA'S HEALTH BENEFITS

Aging: Fungi-melanin, found in the sclerotium (the outside layer of the Chaga) is a powerful anti-aging tool.

Allergies: Medicinal mushrooms (Chaga for one) have super tonic and adaptogenic properties that help fight allergies, asthma and cancer; improve core vitality and helps support a healthy immune system, heart, lungs, kidneys, and lowers elevated blood pressure.

Analgesic: Removes and reduces pain.

Anodyne: Soothes pain.

Antibacterial: Wards off infection and aids in the rapid healing a cut, scrape or burn.

Anti-inflammatory: The compound ergosterol found in Chaga reduces inflammation thus alleviating a bevy of chronic, degenerative diseases, and presumably extending life.

Anti-lipid perxidative: Protects fats from oxidation and loss of electrons.

Anti-oxidant: Reduces sensitivity to painful stimuli.

Anti-parasitic: Removes many types of parasitic worms.

Anti-platelet: Disperses clumped red blood cells.

Anti-tumor: Delays the growth of some kinds of tumors.

Anti-viral: Fights flu, herpes, HIV, and hepatitis.

Arthritis: As an antioxidant is has proved effective in treating arthritis.

Asthma: Alleviates the symptoms associated with asthma and supports good lung health.

Blood Pressure: Lowers arterial and venous blood pressure - improves circulation.

Blood: Purifies the blood and circulatory system.

Brain: Chaga activates the circulation of brain tissue elements and increases bioelectric activity in the cortex of the brain thus improving mental clarity. (as quoted by Robert Rogers, RH (AHG)) [4]

Bronchitis: Strengthens and supports the respiratory system.

Cardio protective: Regulates the heartbeat.

Cancer: Induces apoptosis (spontaneous breakdown of cancer cells) which has a positive effect on the following cancers due to the presence of Beta-Glucan contained in Chaga:

Bone	Medulloblastoma
Breast	Melanoma
Carcinoma	Neuroblastoma
Colon	Ovarian
Hepatoma	Sarcoma
Leukemia	Squamous
Liver	Stomach
Lung	Uterine

Chemotherapy and Radiation: Chaga has proved very effective in supporting standard cancer treatments. It can compensate for the devastating effects these treatments have on the immune system.

Cholesterol: Studies indicate a 50% reduction in glycemic peaks due to the Beta Glucan contained in Chaga, lowering harmful LDL cholesterol.

Cell damage and 'Free radicals': The Chaga contains a powerful anti-oxidant value combating these threats.

Diabetes: Decreases sugar levels in the blood, lowering blood sugar content quickly, and restoring balance.

Heart: By normalizing blood pressure, and cholesterol it contributes to a stronger cardio-vascular system.

Hepatitis C: A recent cell study indicated that Chaga demonstrated a strong activity against this virus.

Herpes: Studies have shown that Chaga reduces the infection due to Herpes simplex virus.

Immune system: The Betulinic acid prevalent in Chaga covers the full range of immune stimulating effects, supporting the immune system.

Intestinal protection: Fights colitis, gastritis, digestive inflammation.

Liver: Purifies and detoxifies.

Nervous system: Calms and eliminates the effects of stress.

Psoriasis: A Russian study concluded that patients who took Chaga experienced a full recovery from psoriasis. This is very significant given that this is notoriously difficult to treat.

Skin, hair and nails: The massive amount of melanin in the Chaga will revitalize these and other organs in the body, giving the user radiant hair, skin, and nails.

Stomach and digestive system: Positively affects stomach disease, ulcers, and improves digestion. The betulinic acid and phytosterols present in the Chaga play an important role in this process.

Sleep: Reduces fatigue and improves sleep.

~ ~ ~ ~ ~ ~

Chaga is a unique, individual being with real science behind it. Scientists have confirmed that no single molecule or property of the Chaga works independently, but rather the sum of all its parts work "intelligently and harmoniously to form a complex 'living medicine'." [5]

Do yourself a huge favor and watch the YouTube presentation by Dr. Karl Maret. [6]

AND THEN THERE'S THAT 3RD EYE THING

The PINEAL Gland

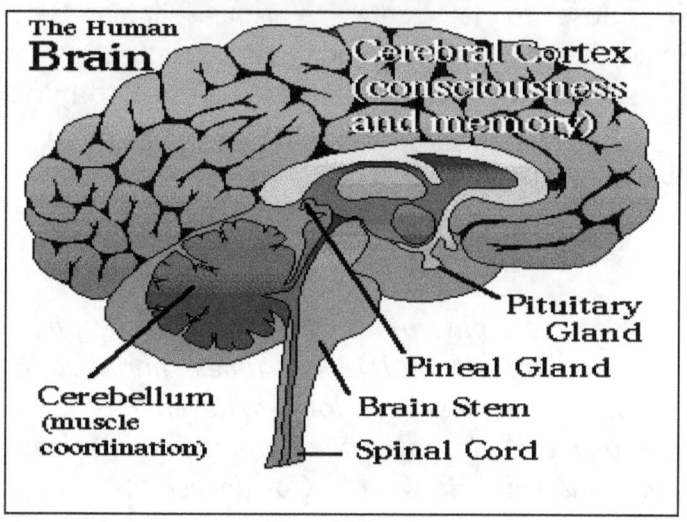

Ahhhh . . . the mystical 'Third Eye."

This important gland was not discovered until late in the evolution of demystifying the functions of the brain. It was not until the 1960s that scientists determined its function, having thought for several decades that it was merely a vestigial organ. (*An organ or structure that has little or no utility, but that in an earlier stage of the individual or in preceding evolutionary forms of the organism performed a useful function like the appendix.*)

Because of our relative ignorance about the pineal gland for so long, it became the object of mythical theories and attributions. Rene Descartes called it the "seat of the soul" because it appeared to be the only brain structure not composed of two symmetrical parts, although later analysis proved this to be untrue. Compounding these rumors was the fact that the pineal gland is lodged very deep within the brain, close to its center. Various shaman-types have claimed that the pineal gland secretes natural psychedelics and is somehow a connection between the earthly realm and a spirit world. These speculations are presumed by science to be likely false.

Pseudoscience Theories

While the physiological function of the pineal gland has been unknown until recent times, mystical traditions and esoteric schools have long believed this area, in the middle of the brain, to be the connecting link between the physical and spiritual worlds. Considered the most powerful and highest source of ethereal energy available to humans, the pineal gland has always been deemed important in initiating supernatural powers. It is believed to control the various bio-rhythms of the body. It works in harmony with the hypothalamus gland which directs the body's thirst, hunger, sexual desire and the biological clock that determines our aging process. When it "awakens", one feels a pressure at the base of the brain. Located deep in the brain it seems to imply a hidden importance. In the days before its function as a physical eye that could see beyond space-time was discovered, it was considered a mystery linked to superstition and mysticism. Today it is associated with the sixth chakra.

The Probable Reality

The medical profession now describes the pineal gland as being: *"a small endocrine gland in the vertebrate brain that produces the serotonin derivative melatonin, a hormone that affects the modulation of wake/sleep patterns and seasonal functions. Its shape resembles a tiny pine cone (hence its name), and it is located near the centre of the brain, between the two hemispheres, tucked in a groove where the two rounded thalamic bodies join."*

Unlike much of the rest of the brain, the pineal gland is not isolated from the body by the blood-brain barrier system. It is reddish-gray and about the size of a pea (8 mm in humans). It is part of the epithalamus. It is a midline structure, and is often seen in plain skull X-rays, as it is frequently calcified. Calcification is typically due to _intake of the fluoride found in water_ _and toothpaste_. It was the last endocrine gland to have its function discovered.

And how does CHAGA affect the Pineal Gland?

According to David Wilcox, likely the world's leading expert on activating the pineal gland, this gland requires melanin to operate at optimum level, and requires more melanin than any other nutrient. Here comes the Chaga, which contains more melanin than any other food or herb known to man. Its nutritional pigments are comparable to those found in the human body.

The addition of melanin, via the Chaga, into ones daily diet will not only promote restorative sleep patterns, improve mental clarity, enhance hair, skin, nails and eyes, and, who knows, it may even tap on the door of the 'mystical world beyond.'

~ ~ ~

[1] *Dr. Ron McDow is a board certified medical doctor of Family Medicine. He attended Medical School at the University Tennessee Center for Health Sciences and*

completed his post graduate training at both the Tennessee Center for Health Sciences and Vanderbilt University Medical Center, where he also studied and received an MBA at Vanderbilt Owen School of Management. He practiced family medicine for 20 plus years before devoting his full time to development of a low cost Cryosurgical Delivery System which was approved by the FDA and patented. Dr. McDow maintains his medical licensure and continues to work in ongoing improvements in the Cryosurgical Delivery System and has developed an interest in uncovering scientifically validated natural nutraceutical products that are not widely recognized or available in Western Medicine.

[2] *Chris Kilham -- Medicine Hunter, Inc. Chris Kilham is a medicine hunter, author and educator. Chris has conducted medicinal field research in over 30 countries. CNN calls Chris "The Indiana Jones of natural medicine." Chris is FOX News' Medicine Hunter and is a regular expert on* The Dr. Oz Show. *He has appeared on* ABC's 20/20, Good Morning America, NBC Nightly News, CNBC's Power Lunch *and CNN Health. He's been featured in* The New York Times, The Wall Street Journal, Psychology Today *and* Outside Magazine.

[3] *Mineral deficiencies are primarily the outcome of the poisoning of our Earth, its atmosphere, and the environment by the excessive use of pesticides, fertilizers, and herbicides, disrupting the food chain, ending up on our dinner plates and pollutants profaning the air we breathe. The further refining and microwaving of our food is another contributing factor. Drugs also interfere with the absorption of minerals, and with age, and lack of exercise, our bodies' ability to replenish these minerals decreases.*

[4] *Robert Rogers, RH (AHG) teaches plant medicine at Grant MacEwan University in Edmonton, Canada. He serves as chair of the medicinal mushroom committee of the North American Mycological Association.*

[5] *From David Wolfe's "CHAGA, King of the Medicinal Mushrooms"*

[6] *Karl Maret, MD, MEng, serves as president of the <u>Dove Health Alliance,</u> and was instrumental in its inception. His broad training as an electrical engineer, biomedical engineer, and medical doctor has given him a solid background in Energy Medicine. He has carried out physiological research at the highest places on earth, including near the summit of Mt. Everest, as well as building specialty instruments for physiological measurements under the Antarctic ice. He has served as a military officer with distinction and run his own consulting business for many years. Prior to serving the Dove Health Alliance he was president of another nonprofit foundation while simultaneously helping hundreds of clients within the field of complementary medicine.*

<u>*Siberian Chaga is neither plant nor animal yet its DNA make up is 30% closer to humans than plants.*</u>

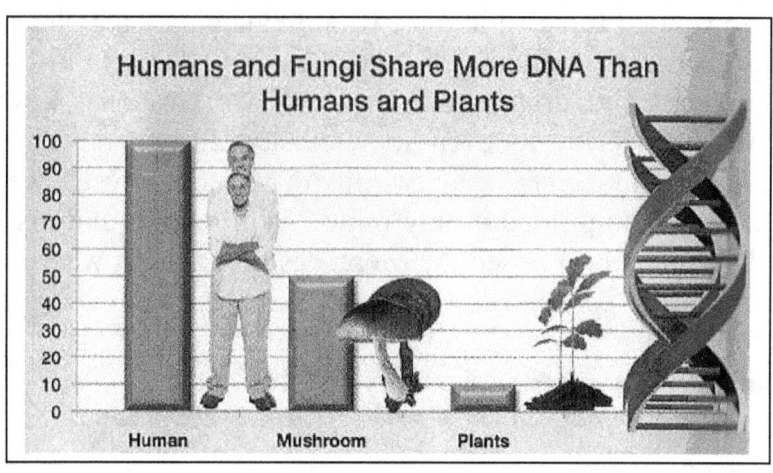

Chapter *Ten*

THE HUNT BEGINS

In the beginning, I teamed up with a buddy of mine who was experiencing a brief sojourn from gainful employment. Billy was a Maine boy, living in Dover Foxcroft, and we had known each other since our early school days. The year was 2010, and I had just stumbled upon the discovery of Chaga --- courtesy of the Mercedes accident and my imposed furlough. With both of us out-of-work, we had plenty of time on our hands to peruse the back roads and trails of the Maine woods.

Billy became a champion Chaga-spotter. While I drove, his keen eyes ferreted out our elusive quarry. We drove over camp roads, logging roads, ATV trails and sometimes --- no roads at all! The 'ole Mercedes 'war-horse' performed like the trouper she was --- *offspring of a John Deere Tractor and a Sherman Tank*. She was nearly indestructible.

Turns out the years I spent, and the experience I gained working as a surveyor with the USGS (United States Geological Survey) in the deep woods of Northern Maine, served me extremely well in this new undertaking. During those years, I traveled into areas impregnable by anyone but the most intrepid hunter or hiker. Having access to hi-tech equipment and driving big Dodge Power wagons, I was privy to a world few even knew existed. Fortunately those trails, and the secret underworld of Maine's forests, were still deeply imprinted on my mind. With daring and just a little trepidation I nosed the Mercedes down paths where no road worthy car, and few off-road vehicles, had ever gone before and we headed toward the famous Forks just a bit south of where we'd broken loose of the forest.

The Forks is known as a snowmobiling and whitewater rafting destination. You can traverse more than 100 miles of interconnected snowmobiling trails that crisscross the region. The Forks is located where the Dead River and Kennebec River meet—making it the starting point for riding these two rivers. Here you can take a 12-mile trip on the Kennebec River trip that begins on Indian Pond and roars through the Upper Kennebec Gorge, with rapids up to class IV. You can also traverse the Dead River, which provides the longest stretch of continuous whitewater in the East.

After moving on from the Forks, we turned our sights on Shirley, Maine. We forged streams and wallowed through gullies, breaking trails where none had been before. Our wheels were frequently entrapped in deep furrows with our underbelly straddling above and being heartily scraped from beneath. We honestly didn't know where we were, but had no doubt that no one else had been on this 'road' for probably a millennium and a half. At best it served as an ATV trail and no way should a full-size vehicle be on it. We looked for a place, any place, to turn ourselves around but none presented themselves and we continued on for what seemed like miles, with the situation growing progressively worse. The 'ole Mercedes hung in there, climbing at times what amounted to be raw ledges where no road seemed to exist anymore.

THE SIEGE OF SHIRLEY

> *Shirley is a town in Piscataquis County, Maine with a population of 233 as recorded on the 2010 census. Incorporated on March 4, 1834, it is the birthplace of humorist Bill Nye --- 'The Science Guy'. It's sweetly set along the Piscataquis River just south of Greenville on 52.9 square miles, and boasts a population density of 4.4 people per square mile.*
> *This is the town we laid siege to . . .*

With relief we spied sunlight ahead and with great delight we broke through the underbrush and burst out into an open field. *The Mercedes had safely got us back to civilization.* However as our car broke through the dense forest's plumage and we plunged forth onto the town square of Shirley, we set off quite a commotion. Two old geezers sittin' and rockin' on the porch of the town's small general store 'bout had a heart attack! Never . . . in all their memory did they ever see (or expect to see) a full-grown car, with two crazed men on board, come barrelin' hell-bent out of the forest on an ATV trail!

Well, after we had done some visiting and settled all the town folk down, convincing them that we were not conquistadors from some invading country to the North, we gathered ourselves together and nosed the 'ole Mercedes north toward Moosehead Lake. Fortunately, I remembered from my surveying days, an old logging road that could take us all the way to Moosehead Lake. That was our goal and once we were on it, found it to be a rather easy road to traverse. Not to continue as such! The road deteriorated rapidly as we proceeded north and we soon realized that we were on what amounted to another ATV trail. Still, for the moment, this seemed to present no problem for the Mercedes. We headed north!

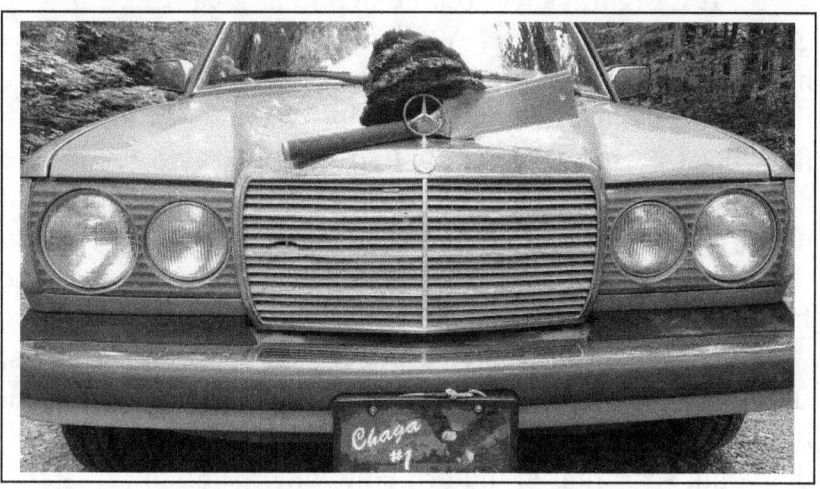

This jaunt made me recall another hunt when I was all by myself heading toward Eagle Lake. It had rained a good deal prior to my jaunt and the backwood roads were in deplorable condition (nearly non-existent). I drove mile after mile in conditions that truly taxed both me and the ole' Mercedes. It made me question my sanity. But I survived, and to the amazement of my auto mechanic he could scarcely believe the old girl was still running after all the abuse she'd suffered through.

Now it might sound as though these Chaga hunts were all about the primordial conditions that we 'boys' put ourselves through - kinda' like a 'coming-of-age' ritual from boys to men. My wife might agree with that theory but the truth is we collected a lot of Chaga on these hair-raising expeditions. Once harvested, the Chaga was stowed in the back seat in paper bags, which allowed them to breathe and slowly dry out. The drying-out process is of great importance in protecting and sustaining the integrity of the valued nutrients of this amazing mushroom. It must be accomplished as quickly as possible as it can be attacked by other fungi.

It is significance to note here that great care must be given to the host tree. A Chaga can - and should - be harvested with the minimal trauma to its host. There are those who believe it best to use only bare hands to remove the Chaga. I use a tool but apply it with the same gentle care a surgeon might employ when operating upon a patient under his knife.   Each Chaga hunter has an opinion regarding the best time of year to harvest these gems. The fall and winter seasons certainly make the Chaga more visible, for the leaves have dropped, snow covers the forest floor and swathes bare tree limbs. It is in this environment that the Chaga appears to glow like an iridescent black diamond, sparkling in the brilliant winter sunlight. It is also theorized by some that because in winter the tree is dormant and the sap not running, that the Chaga is at its most potent peak. However, I find the most agreeable seasons for hunting are during the warm months of late summer and early fall. True, the Chaga is more difficult to seek out but the hunt is so much more pleasant when your teeth aren't chattering and you're not experiencing chilblains. I also question whether the Chaga is indeed more potent when the sap has ceased flowing. The Chaga is made up of a hard woody sponge-like material that has been soaking up and absorbing the trees nutrients for decades. The change of season and the cessation of the sap flow would have no effect upon it, and in fact, a winter harvest could be contrary to the well-being of the tree for even when appearing dormant the tree is supplying its nutrients to the Chaga.

Think of the Hippocratic Oath: "First do no harm."

I feel it is vitally important to caution all who seek out, and harvest, the Chaga that the methods used greatly effect the host tree and its parasitic gift. It benefits the continued growth of the Chaga to take only a segment of the Chaga, leaving a goodly portion of it on the tree to assure its continued growth, and it's possible to mark the tree with your GPS and return to the same tree a year later to harvest a bit more. With each harvesting of the Chaga I'm very careful not to cut into the tree itself and by doing so the bit that remains will harden over and continue to grow for the life of the tree. Unfortunately, the white birch has only a life-span of 50 to 60 years (unlike those of its neighbor, the oak tree). To find birches of that age you must go deep into the northern climes where the trees thrive best in the extreme sub-zero temperatures. If we do not become stewards of our forests and this precious mushroom, it will surely become extinct, if not in our lifetime, then certainly the next. I'm already observing birches in the northern New England states that appear in dire straits. The signs are already out there. Global warming perhaps?

As mentioned earlier, it is of extreme importance that the Chaga be properly dried out immediately. It should be set out in strong sunlight until totally dry, and before any fungus can attack it, then stored in a manner that assures proper air circulation and ventilation.

A method I've often found very effective, when traveling with my kayak strapped right-side-up on the roof of the Mercedes, is to stow the harvested Chaga securely wrapped inside a pillowcase into the bed of the up-turned kayak. The combination of air-flow and concentrated sunlight pouring down as I drive about the North Country does a superb job of curing.

Aside from the care a Chaga hunter must practice, the hunter must also cultivate extreme patience, for some days there are no sightings, and even weeks can go by without a smidgen of a hint of the elusive quarry. A full season of harvesting might total a yield of just 30 to 40 pounds of product. It has been estimated that out of a possible 20,000 birch trees, there may be just 20 useable, proper sized and harvest-ready Chaga. A hunter must find irresistible the lure of woodlands, the solitude, and being one-with-nature, for the rewards of the hunt may just be a bit underwhelming.

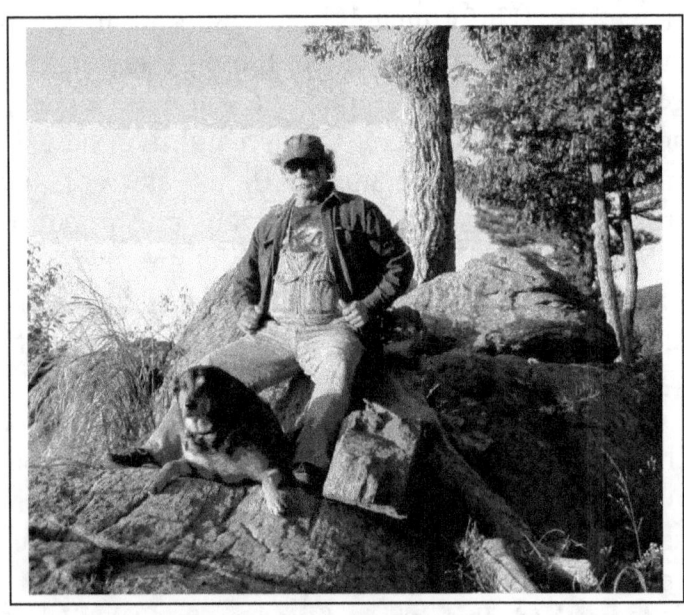

Chapter *Eleven*

The Revolution ~ The Evolution ~ and Burt and I

The 60's. Haight-Ashbury. This was the time and the place to be young, to be alive and to be part of a movement to change the world. The message, the music, the flowers and, yes, even the drugs, were the allure of the movement. The youth of our nation, and of the world, had cast to the winds the straight-jacketed lives and ideals of their middle-class parents, and the boorish political dogma of the establishment. The media hyped it, labeling it the "Hippie Movement". Stuffed-shirted executives abhorred it, parents feared it, and song-writers sang about it. Jefferson Airplane, the Mamas & the Papas, the Grateful Dead, and Janis Joplin were just a few who immortalized it with a new musical genre called "psychedelic rock". Eventually, a hit stage musical was borne of it called "Hair".

It began with the "Flower Children", a new breed of young people who wanted to be in tune with their spirituality, with nature, and with the universe. Others from all walks of life began to heed the message, wanted to be part of it, and thus began the migration west to the "City of Love," San Francisco. Like an overpowering tornado, it sucked the best, the bravest, the more adventurous, and most idealistic of America's youth into its vortex. By 1967 there were 100,000 teenagers, college students, runaways, a smattering of the military, and even a few curious vacationers drawn into this cultural phenomenon. Then came its implosion. Soft drugs became hard drugs. Homelessness, hunger, overcrowding, and crime infected this utopian spawning ground. The *Grand Experiment* had failed. On October 6, 1967 those few remaining at Haight-Ashbury staged a mock funeral with the following eulogy:

> *"We wanted to signal that this*
> *was the end of it, don't come out.*
> *Stay where you are! Bring the*
> *revolution to where you live.*
> *Don't come here because it's*
> *over and done with."*

But the "revolution" hadn't died. Instead, it was broadcasted far and wide across this vast country by every idealized kid that had lived, breathed, and believed in the message of Haight-Ashbury. Communities and communes sprang up where none had been before; throughout middle-America, up and down the west coast, the eastern seaboard, and straight to New York's Greenwich Village. It was a valiant attempt to regain that 'spark', to get back to nature, to reignite their connection to the universe, to nurture their spirituality, and to recapture those ideals that had triggered the movement to Haight-Asbury.

One such place of migration was Summertown, Tennessee where 'hippie' Stephen Gaskin pioneered a communal-lifestyle community. This is known as *The Farm and* still exists today as a strong and healthy community with families living close to the land and home-schooling their children.

Scott and Helen Nearing are another example of this "counter-culture" revolution having 'dropped out' of society in the 1940's to create a simple back-to-nature life in Vermont. They later recaptured it in Cape Rosier Maine, where their memory is cherished to this day, and their followers still live and flourish. The Nearings wrote books about their life style, and were often featured in "Mother Earth" magazine, and as a result, many of those who migrated from Haight-Ashbury to the northeast, became followers of the Nearings.

This brings me to a unique fellow, an offshoot of Haight-Ashbury, who eventually ended up in my part of the world; Dover-Foxcroft, Maine. His name was Burt and he sold honey. At that time I was living in a sweet little cabin beside a spring, while Burt contentedly existed in an abandoned chicken coop (yes- a chicken coop) somewhere in the general vicinity. He had become a bee-keeper, maintaining a good size apiary of about 50 bee hives, and was making a modest living selling his honey in town from the back of his truck, which he had painted 'school bus' yellow to attract customers. Burt - last name Shavitz was a bit of a recluse and very content to live humbly, forgoing the 'niceties' that his fellowman required.

Now these were the days of safe hitch-hiking, and the highways and byways were frequently teaming with guys and gals, thumbs out, begging a ride. On one spring day while traveling home Burt stopped and offered a pretty gal a lift. Her name was Roxanne. This seemingly random act of chivalry, for Roxanne Quimby, was to change Bert's life forever, as she had entered his life to stay.

Roxanne, with true Yankee entrepreneurial spirit, was not content to live in a chicken coop, and saw the potential of creating a business from the excess beeswax of Burt's operation. She began experimenting and her first creation was lip balm. She began marketing it in small round tins and labeling it "Burt's Bees Lip Balm." She, the aggressive entrepreneur, and Burt, the mellow laid-back recluse, became partners and continued making, and selling, candles and lip balm at the local farmers markets. Their business took off - from an initial $200.00 gleaned at a junior-high school fair, to $20,000 at the end of their first year of operation. This subsequently changed their life-style, and they moved their business into an abandoned one-room schoolhouse. There, Roxanne continued experimenting successfully with other marketable creations derived from beeswax. The rest is history.

Soon Burt's Bees Inc. featured, not only candles, but over 100 natural personal-care products, and his brand, with his face upon it, had become famous world-wide.

Fame, and all the hoopla that trails in its wake, was not Burt's 'cuppa tea'. He remained a singularly antisocial character, an eccentric, avoiding people and all their random conversation. His mantra: "A good day is when no one shows up and you don't have to go anywhere. I get four channels - spring, summer, fall, and winter from right outside my window"

(Check out *Burt's Buzz* on YouTube)

In time, fame and fortune overwhelmed poor Burt. All he ever wanted from life was peace, quiet and to be left alone. Suddenly he finds himself flying all over the world, conducting seminars, and promoting the products that Roxanne was producing from his humble bee apiary. The company became so huge and unwieldy that it outgrew its home base in Maine and it was moved to North Carolina. Eventually the business partnership between he and Roxanne soured, and he was forced out of his own company. Ultimately, Burt's Bees was sold to the CLOROX Company for a figure somewhere in the vicinity of $300,000,000. Burt returned to Maine and to his "chicken coop", though improvements had been made to it; electricity, a telephone, and a FAX machine added. Once returned to his reclusive seclusion he built a proper home for Roxanne so that she might live in comparable comfort. It is reputed that he loved the lady 'til the day he died. His face still appears on Burt's Bees products and for that, he received a stipend of $40,000 quarterly until his death in 2015.

~ ~ ~ ~ ~ ~

So it was a bit out of character (and a remarkable perk for me) that he and I met, chatted, and established a friendship of sorts.

Before the fame and fortune entered Burt's life, both he and I were living it close proximity to the sleepy little town of Dexter, Maine, where resided a smattering of neighborhood pubs. One that I often frequented was *Rubin's Glo,* and while there I began to notice an old guy sitting alone, and away from all possible human contact. I suspected he was an introvert of some kind, sipping on his glass of red wine, and avoiding all eye contact with fellow bar patrons. I got up my courage one day, approached him, and struck up a conversation (I now know this was an agonizing exchange for Burt to participate in). However, he and I connected at some level, perhaps from the dust of our Haight-Ashbury days, and we eventually became friends.

Burt was an animal lover in the extreme and owned a beautiful golden retriever named Rufus, which he absolutely adored. At that time my dog Tia, a shepherd/lab mix, had just delivered a litter of nine puppies. Well, Burt couldn't resist the lure of a bevy of puppies, and he began to visit my cabin on a regular basis to play with these little guys and our friendship grew.

~ ~ ~ ~ ~ ~ ~

As life would have it our paths took us in different directions Then, some years later Burt and I bumped into each other again at a place called the *Wagon Wheel Bar*, a seasonal Maine establishment, open only during hunting season. When Burt entered the bar and saw me, he immediately invited me to come outside, see his new car and to have a visit with Rufus. He had bought a magnificent pearl-white 1985 Mercedes station wagon, and had it brought directly from Germany! It was furnished complete with a mattress in the back, so that he and Rufus could sleep in it while touring the countryside. Though Bert's Bees had provided him with the funds to purchase such a superb vehicle, he still shunned comfort and followed his wanderlust spirit.

Well, I had just discovered the Chaga mushroom, and was deep into studying the many potential benefits it offered. I shared this information with Burt and we chatted about my ideas to further investigate the Chaga and possibly develop a product from it, one which I could market that would enhance folk's wellbeing. I was considering beginning with a simple concoction, a beneficial healing balm. And so I asked Burt . . .

"Burt," I said "I don't want to compete with you, your success, or your many products, but if you could steer me in the right direction, and answer just one simple question for me, I'd be eternally grateful. What do you think would be the simplest product for me to create, and what should I use for a base?"

He answered simply, "A healing balm. Shea butter."*

And with that simple advice I was on my way to developing Golden Chaga Balm, my first product and an exceptional healing balm.

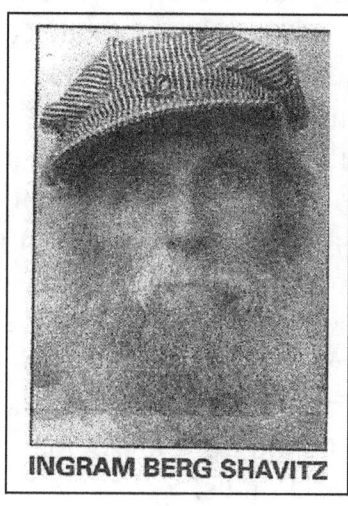

INGRAM BERG SHAVITZ

When I returned to Florida I wanted to test the validity of this, my first product, and I passed out samples to friends and relatives, urging them to try it. The very first success that I was able to document was that of my neighbor Bob. He had developed a receding hairline coupled with numerous pre-cancerous skin lesions on his scalp. Thus far he had been treated with 3 laser skin peels, a treatment which had proved to be very painful, and offered him no apparent solution. So I suggested he give the Chaga balm a try. He did, and three weeks later he and his wife visited us and he showed me his scalp. Sure enough, his scalp was covered with new skin ("Like a baby's bottom") and there were no more lesions. He was excited, and vehemently encouraged me to "get going and market this stuff." Of course, that had long been the plan at the back of my mind. So enthusiastic was he that he offered to build a website for me (the website wouldn't happen until sometime later), and help to get the word out about this marvelous new product.

I promised that I would certainly consider this proposal and that Terry and I would discuss it further.

On the heels of that chat, Terry and I agreed to meet with Bob and his wife and explore the possibilities over dinner. While Terry was driving us to their home, over one of Florida's back roads, I got a call from my friend Mike, and as I was talking to him I realized the car had suddenly stopped. I looked at Terry and saw she was pointing, wide-eyed, to a huge bald eagle in the middle of the road! And as we watched two other eagles joined him. As they were effectively blocking the road, we were privy to an extended sighting of these magnificent birds. It made quite an impact on us.

Some weeks later, I related this event to a friend of mine, who is of Native-American descent. His response to our sighting truly convinced us that we were on the right track, and should move forward with our fledgling Chaga business. His interpretation of this unusual sighting? Those three eagles appearing before us was a sign of *"very powerful medicine"* and an indication that something of significance was about to befall us.

That evening after dinner and following the eagle sighting, we solidified our plans and Golden Chaga was born!

And so it was that my youthful affiliation with Haight-Ashbury opened the doorway to an unprecedented friendship with recluse Bert Shavitz, and climaxed by the power of three bald eagles, led me to the creation of a new and marvelous business enterprise, GOLDEN CHAGA. Thus began the amazing journey of a lifetime.

* Shea butter comes from the nut of a tree that grows in Africa. When the nut is harvested, it is crushed, then boiled and the oils that rise to the top are what we know as shea butter.

Chapter *Twelve*

POTPOURRI

A little bit of this and some of that.

There are many tales and events that have flowed in and out of my life, and influenced my quest for the Chaga; this may be a good place to relate a few of them.

FAMOUS HEALER

There is a history in my family of a healer, a healer of a very unique kind. My great, great, great grandmother was Mary Foster Burke. She was born in Liverpool, Nova Scotia, in 1763 and lived for a remarkable 88 years, spending her entire life among the Mic-Mac Indians. She was regarded by them as the "Messenger of The Great Spirit" due to her remarkable powers to heal and cure the sick, and she is reputed to be the first white woman to serve as mid-wife among the Indian tribes of North America. Her prowess in administrating to the sick lay in her ability to know, and seek out, the powerful healing herbs and native plants that abound in the North Country. No one knows today just how well acquainted with medicine, in the modern sense of the word, Mrs. Burke was, but it has definitely been established that she doctored her patients with natural herbs, and always with amazing results.

In times of need, Indians from near and far sought her services, for her fame as a healer had spread throughout the wilderness. Special parties were sent to transport her to various destinations to perform her healing rites. Anything she needed was immediately provided to her.

Though I have no proof, I firmly believe that the Chaga was no doubt, one of the chosen natural curatives she utilized to affect the many cures she is reputed to have facilitated.

Because of her untiring and devoted service to the Mic-Macs, and all the tribes of the North Country whom she looked upon as equals, she was highly regarded by them, and was treated like royalty. She and her husband were provided with fresh venison, fish, fruits and berries harvested from the forests and waters by their devoted Indian neighbors on an ongoing basis.

(This account was drawn from an interview with C. Foster Lambert - great, great grandson of Mrs. Burke (and my great granduncle)) - written by Kalil Ayoob, and published in the Bangor Daily News - Bangor, Maine ~1842)

APPARENTLY IT RUNS DEEP WITHIN MY FAMILY

I made the mistake of mentioning to the lady who is writing this book that TOM'S OF MAINE was a distant cousin of mine through marriage.

"WHAT!" she said. "That needs to be mentioned in this book. The products that he and his company have developed are true assets to the world. I used the stuff myself!"

So, under extreme pressure, we're adding a bit about "cousin" Tom. Here's the skinny.

All products: body lotions & washes, deodorants & antiperspirants, lip balms & soap, toothpaste & baby products are made with only natural ingredients. They contain no phthalates, parabens or phenoxy ethanol.

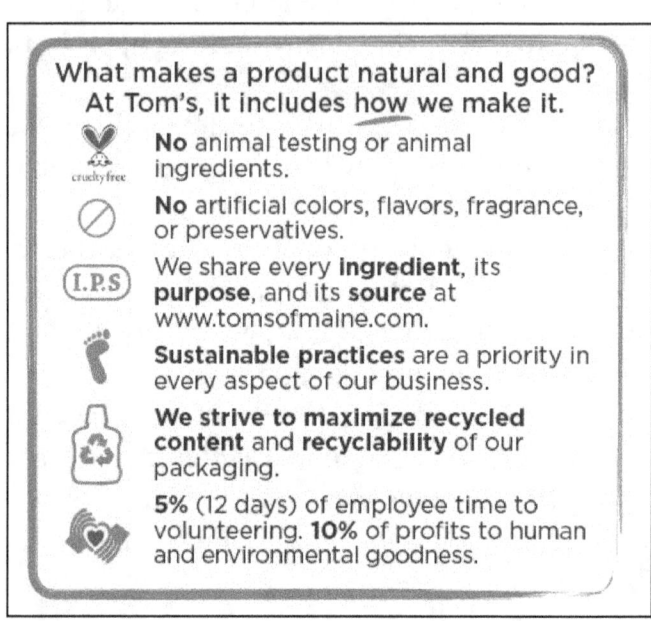

Founded in 1970 by Tom and Kate Chapell with just $5000, products manufactured by the Kennebunk, Maine, firm are sold at more than 40,000 retail outlets worldwide. Their global outreach began in 2006 when Tom's of Maine became a partially owned subsidiary of Colgate-Palmolive. The reason for this highly successful enterprise is that aside from making money, this company has retained its core values which are detailed in Tom's 1994 book, "The Soul of a Business: Managing for Profit and the Common Good"

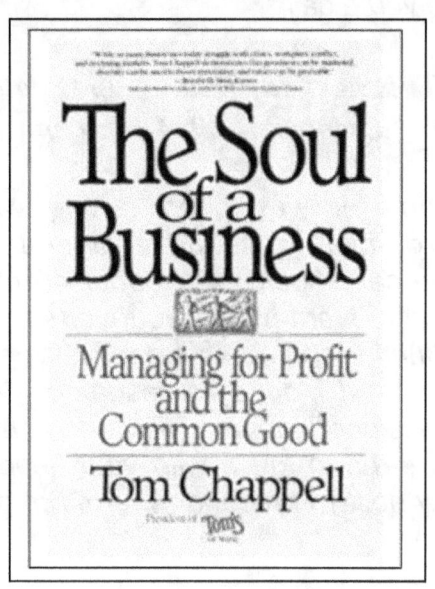

AND THEN, I ALMOST BECAME A TELEVISION CELEBRITY

The following is taken directly from a media inquiry dated October 6, 2014- 1:14 pm.

"Hi Golden Chaga, My name is Molly Sebastian and I am currently a Casting Director working in Development with ITV Studios. ITV Studios is a full scale, International production company responsible for many hit series including The First 48 on A&E, Four Weddings on TLC and Kitchen Nightmares on FOX.

We are currently working on a project for a network and we are looking for people that have a job where it is required that you brave the elements and work outside, sometimes in brutally cold, treacherous conditions and where there is a risk/reward quotient. We are especially interested in Chaga Hunters.

If you are interested in talking, please email your number and I will give you a call."

This next day follow- up is dated
October 7, 2014 - 2:02pm

"Hi Barry! It was good talking with you. As I mentioned, I'd love to set-up a time to do a Skype interview. The call should take about 45 minutes and it's our opportunity to learn more about you and your business and Chaga Hunting. I am pasting my Skype tips below. I'd love to aim for next Monday, Tuesday or Wednesday and whatever time is good for you, will work for me.
Also, I'd love to be in touch with your nephew. Please let me know how best to proceed in terms of getting in touch with him."

Alas, it was not to be. The focus of their intended programming was simply not a good fit for me. They were seeking a "reality-type" format rather than one of supporting the environment, conservation, forestry management, and that of the universal benefits of the Chaga.

Chapter *Thirteen*

AND SO IT BEGINS

Once Burt steered me on the right path, I was 'up-and-running' - and *GOLDEN CHAGA* was born!

Golden Chaga was established to promote and market the various products we planned to produce from the miraculous gift of the birch tree.

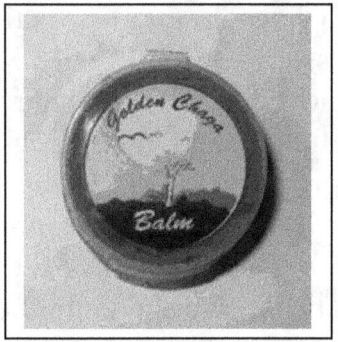

ONE: Chaga Balm was the first product and prepared with a base of shea butter, just as Burt had advised. This balm is used topically with pretty amazing results.

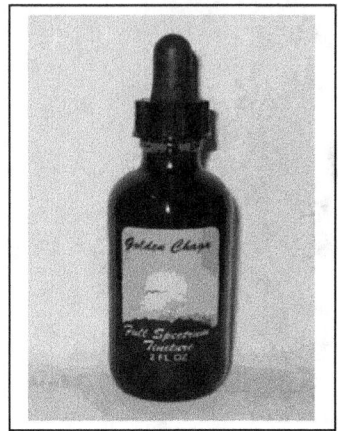

TWO: Then we turned our attention to researching future products, and quickly discovered that the full spectrum tincture was the most revered, world wide, of all of its derivates. This liquid is applied by placing a small amount of it under the tongue, letting it mix with the saliva, and finally allowing it to dissolve into the minuscule blood vessels beneath the tongue. This method of application is referred to as sublingual, its results are almost immediate, and the benefits are many. To achieve the full spectrum benefits, which include all the nutrients known to be in the Chaga, a dual extraction process is utilitized. This process was used in early Russia and the technique is still employed today. The end result is known and promoted as befungin and used specifically in the cancer wards of Eastern Europe.

So now, *Golden Chaga* has two products: Chaga Balm for external healing and the Full Spectrum Tincture -used internally, and benefiting the entire body. We were on our way!

Our next step was to look into the possibilities of products for face and body.

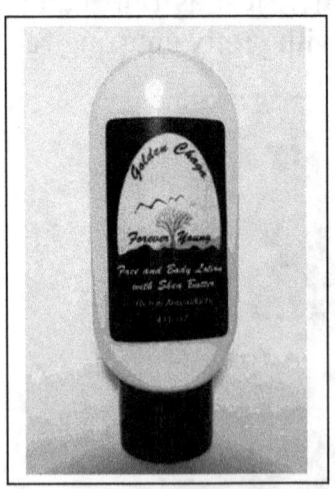

THREE: It is a known fact that Chaga is the richest source of melanin in the world. It is also a known fact that melanin is the most important nutrient for healthy skin, hair, nails and eyes. It is a sad fact that with the advent of aging the body's natural ability to produce melanin declines. This triggers other maladies of the aging process and a whole 'laundry list' of degenerative diseases. As the body's natural production of melanin slows down, the all-important pineal gland suffers. This gland functions as the 'control center' for the endocrine system which in turn helps to create a strong, balanced immune system. Therefore, with the decline of its natural melanin production the entire body suffers. So I felt it was important to create a lotion for the external body, the skin. The skin is the body's largest organ and most absorptive. Everything we place upon this organ ultimately ends up within our entire system.

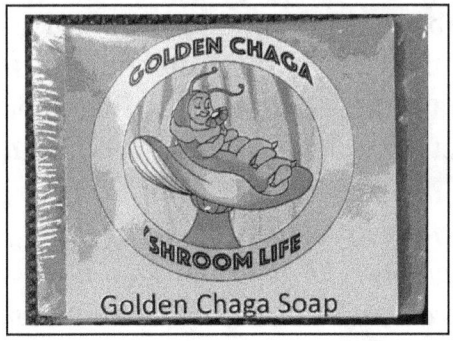

Golden Chaga Soap

FOUR: I'm convinced that my next product came to me in a dream, and with that dream still fresh in my head; I contacted Sarah from New Jersey. She is a retired bio chemist who began an all-natural soap company, the finest in Central Florida. I asked her if she could concoct a soap product if I provided her with the concentrated

Chaga extract. Well, she agreed and Golden Chaga Soap quickly became one of our most popular products.

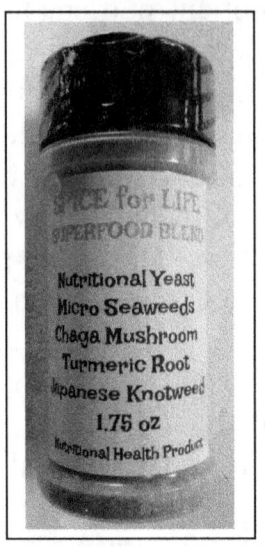

FIVE: Recently, there has been a lot of hype about 'superfoods' and the burgeoning industries being created around and about, these products. One such informational presentation that caught my attention was broadcast on one of the major networks expounding upon the future of these products. *(Superfoods are a special category of foods found in nature. By definition they are calorie sparse and nutrient dense meaning they pack a lot of punch for their weight as far as goodness goes. They are superior sources of anti-oxidants and essential nutrients, nutrients we need but cannot make ourselves.)*

Well, our next creation seemed to be a no-brainer. The benefits of the Chaga, with its vast nutritional attributes, appeared to be a perfect fit for a superfood product. Armed with that knowledge, I conceived our next product: SPICE for LIFE - A Superfood Blend, which comes in its own shaker for ease of sprinkling on foods, just like a salt and pepper shaker! This 'spice' is a blend of all my favorite superfoods: Nutritional Yeast, Micro Seaweeds, Chaga Mushroom, Turmeric Root and Japanese Knotweed. These are all very powerful antioxidants.

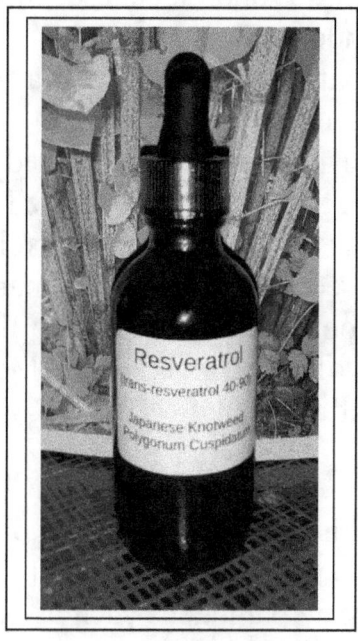

NOT A CHAGA PRODUCT
(But a very important addition
to the health and wellbeing of mankind.)
RESVERATROL

SIX: Unrelated to any of my Chaga products, is one that I have added to my repertoire and known as reseveratrol. This is a superfood derived from a plant that arrived in this country near the turn of the century, and was viewed mainly as an ornamental offering. Like so many foreign 'visitors' it escaped into our environment, invading the northeast. I began researching this plant, which I now know to be Japanese Knotweed, and found it to be the richest known source of reseveratrol. This "invasive weed" is the key 'vessel' to this highly effective product. It had been used for centuries in Chinese and Japanese medicines as an effective life extender.

I discovered that many before me had researched the Japanese Knotweed, and with amazing results. These results, compiled by much respected doctors and scientists, had been generously shared by any who wished to access the information. Excited at having discovered this weed and its very remarkable benefits and attributes, I took my information to the Agricultural Extension Office of the University of Maine where my findings were confirmed.

~ ~ ~ ~ ~ ~

Resveratrol is a stilbenoid, a type of natural phenol and a phytoalexin produced naturally by several plants when under attack by pathogens such as bacteria or fungi – especially the roots of the Japanese Knotweed. These are thought to act like antioxidants, protecting the body against damage that can put it at higher risk for cancer and heart disease. It is believed to be extremely beneficial for the following maladies:

Heart disease: It's thought to help reduce inflammation, lower LDL or "bad" cholesterol, and make it more difficult for clots to form that can lead to a heart attack.

Cancer: It could limit the spread of cancer cells and start killing them.

111

Alzheimer's: It may protect nerve cells from damage and fight the plaque buildup that can lead to the disease.

Diabetes: Resveratrol helps prevent insulin resistance, a condition in which the body becomes less sensitive to the blood sugar-lowering hormone insulin. The condition can lead to diabetes.

Bone Health and Osteoporosis: Resveratrol is very beneficial in the stimulation of bone formation.

Researchers also believe that resveratrol activates the SIRT1 gene the gene that is believed to protect the body against the effects of obesity and the diseases of aging.

~ ~ ~ ~ ~ ~

Armed with my new-found knowledge I began gathering the roots of this plant from the pristine mountains of Maine. I dried them and processed them by means of a very ancient Chinese method - utilizing rice vinegar - thereby extracting the reseveratrol from the Knotweed.

~ ~ ~ ~ ~ ~

Now with five products, plus the reseveratrol, I felt armed with enough product, and information, to go forth and market these beneficial offerings to mankind.

THE GOLDEN CHAGA LOGO

In Lewis Carroll's book of *Alice in Wonderland,* there has always been a question about just what was the caterpillar Absolem was smoking in that hookah pipe. Do a bit of research, and it will leave you scratching your head, for none of the 'experts' on the life of Lewis Carroll will agree on this topic. Was it simply tobacco - or *something else?* So dear reader I will leave this matter up to you and your own imagination. However, as I loved the image of the caterpillar lounging blissfully upon a mushroom, and seemingly reaping the blissful benefits of (possible) Chaga usage, I chose to modify this theme and adapt it as my logo. Ultimately, Alyssa, the daughter of a friend of mine, created this design (minus the hookah and adding a sweet little flower instead) and we've used it ever since. For me it implies a good life, a healthy life, a long life, and a life filled with peace and serenity.

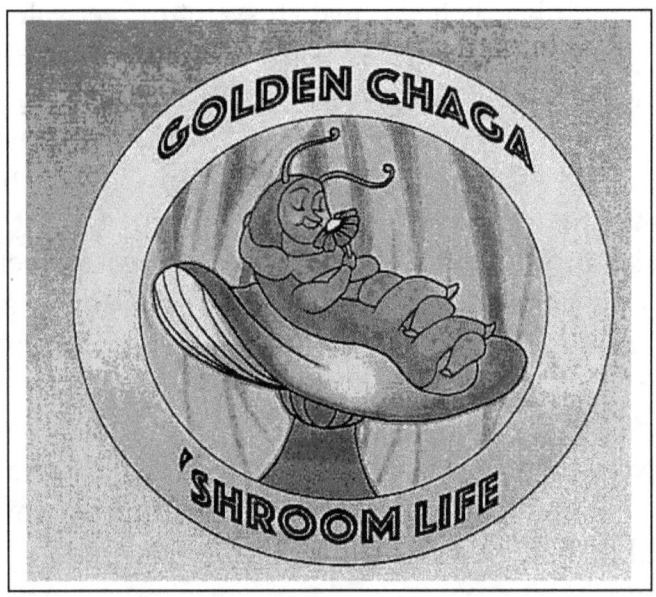

NOW FOR THE MARKETING

We knew it would be a tough sell. We knew its' success rested fully upon the education of the general public, and their willingness to devote a few minutes to hear us out.

Our first foray into the world of marketing was at a small flea market in Oakhill, Florida. Our display booth consisted of a table, with a canopy above, and our products displayed prominently among various pieces of literature and books, and, of course, our Golden Chaga logo waving bravely over all. The books, of course, touted the virtues of the Chaga, and were written by the many current experts in the field.

Well, no surprise, not only were the attendees disinterested in us and our products, but appeared totally suspicious of what we were marketing.

"Mushrooms, huh?"

"Yeah, I've heard of them mushrooms. Kinda 'Magic' huh?"

"Hey man, what kind of trip will these take me on?"

Oh . . . harkening back to the sixties. We heard them all, and as people passed us by it seemed to us that they would purposely avert their eyes, and gaze off into some far distant horizon, so as not to be caught glancing at a product that seemed to them a scant chary, and maybe even a bit illegal.

But we hung in there, and slowly folks did stop to listen, and learn, and even ventured to buy a product or two. This was encouraging, for many of these folks would return the following month to buy more, and relate the positive ways in which Chaga had changed their lives.

Occasionally someone would stop by who knew about Chaga and was delighted to find it here in Florida. Usually these were 'snow-birds' or vacationers from northern New England, regions where Chaga is harvested and therefore better known.

And so we moved forward, adding more venues and outlets to our itinerary which included the Volusia County Fair Ground's weekly "Farmer's Market". This particular market has grown far beyond the typical farmer's market, currently boasting over 400 venders selling every imaginable item, from native-grown foodstuffs to eclectic treasures recycled from someone's trash bin and so much more.

At this venue we befriended Stuart, a successful vendor of trash bin finds, and here I will relate his story:

His lady-friend, Dawn, had recently been diagnosed with an inoperable tumor, and had been admitted into a Hospice facility, to await her impending demise. This tumor was located in her mouth and lodged deep within her jaw. Its very location generated excruciating pain, as well as preventing any life-saving surgery. As a last-ditch effort Stuart brought her a bottle of Chaga Tincture, which she began applying daily to the tumorous area, holding it in her mouth, and allowing her body to absorb it sublingually.

A couple of months later, when I'm just about ready to head back up to Maine for my annual Chaga harvest, Stuart approached my booth and reported that Dawn's tumor has shrunk. I congratulated him on this small step toward her wellness and he purchased another bottle to take to her. Shortly thereafter, I left for Maine and in my absence Terry continued to set up our booth and promote Chaga at our many venues.

While deep in the forests of Maine, Terry and I always attempt to make contact on a somewhat regular basis. Sometime this works, sometimes not, dependant upon the depth of whatever forest I am currently foraging in. On one such call she informed me that Dawn's tumor had shrunk sufficiently enough for her to move it about with her tongue, and she wondered if she should attempt to pull it out. Terry advised her not to do that but let Chaga, and nature, take its course.

Several months later, with my Maine harvest completed for the year, I returned to Florida and joined Terry on our marketing circuit. It was while back at the Volusia Fair Grounds that Stuart approached us, this time holding a small glass vial in his hand, and through the glass we could see this ugly, nasty-looking thing. "Look," he exclaimed, "this is all that remains of the tumor that was in Dawn's mouth. She's CURED! They kicked her out of Hospice!" (She remains tumor-free to this day. See her personal commentary in chapter 19).

As time went on (it has been 7 years now) more and more people recognized Chaga and know of its virtues. I'm told that even Dr. Oz dedicated a segment of one of his shows to it. (I believe it was *Chris Kilham,* mentioned in chapter 9 that did the presentation).

While at our booth in New Smyrna I was approached by a lady who was seeking Chaga capsules. She had been valiantly battling breast cancer quite successfully with natural herbs and plants, primarily oil of frankincense, and believed that Chaga would fire the final volley to her finish off her cancer. I explained to her that Terry and I had attempted to produce capsules, but with very frustrating results. It may be a simply task for a huge manufacturing company to mechanically stuff medicinal powders into a minuscule opening in a tiny vial and cap it, but the do-it-yourself method makes it nearly impossible. So Terry and I had given up on this. I explained this to the lady and suggested she search the internet for these capsules. Well in doing so, she discovered and related to us that one of the most respected purveyors of the 'Chaga family', a very knowledgeable and respected gentleman from Maine, had had his entire operations investigated by the FDA (Federal Drug Association). This scared the heck out of all of us who hunt and vend Chaga, so I got in touch with my webmaster and he immediately shut down my website. (More about the inequities of this ongoing eyeball-to-eyeball standoff with the FDA in a later chapter.) My webmaster guy was thoroughly incensed by the total unfairness of it all. "The public needs to know about this stuff." was his battle cry. "If you can't safely publicize your message over the internet, then how about doing it in a book?"

I thought that was one heck-of-an-idea!

It just so happened that recently I'd set up a booth in DeLeon Springs, right next to a lady who'd been transplanted to Florida all the way from magnificent (her word) New Hampshire. She was an artist and a writer. We had chatted throughout the day-long event and discovered that we had both lived at one time in Castine, Maine, and although our paths hadn't cross, we knew many of the same people. I had purchased one of her books *"A Sitting Ovation",* which was a compilation of everything she had ever written, both that which had been previously published in New England magazines and periodicals and those which had simply languished in a file cabinet for years. That book was on my bedside table and each night

I'd read a little bit. I liked her style. Soon after my friend challenged me to produce a book I woke suddenly, in the middle of the night, and realized that *I knew a writer!* Fortunately, I'd kept her business card, and I called her the next day to inquire if she would consider ghost-writing a book with me. We met shortly thereafter at the Boston Coffee House in DeLand, and agreed to a writing partnership. (You'll see her name on the front of this book)

~ ~ ~ ~ ~ ~ ~

Do you know that Chaga is good for your pets as well? If you love them, augment their diet with a drop or two of the Chaga Full Spectrum Tincture. (The amount you give them should be determined by their weight)

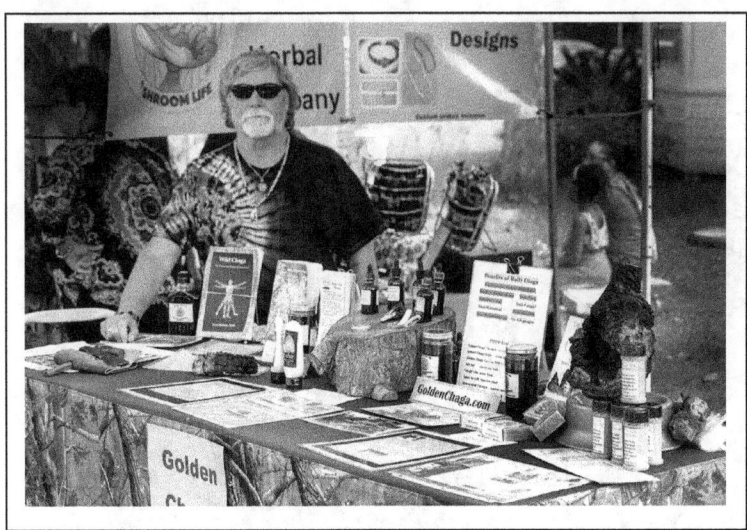

Chapter *Fourteen*

Rainbow Springs - Part I

As I noted in an earlier chapter, Rainbow Springs, an important stop along the Appalachian Trail, was made infamous in the book *"A Walk in the Woods"*, written by Bill Bryson, and later turned into a movie starring Robert Redford. It's true that when Bill stayed there, the conditions of the campground offered an amusing bit of light comedic action to his tale. But that was some years prior to my becoming involved in the management and upkeep of this magnificent spot along the trail.

I discovered Rainbow Springs in 1995 while on a section hike with Charlie (see chapter 6) from Springer Mountain, Georgia, to Clingmans Dome in the Smokies.

"It was love at first sight!"

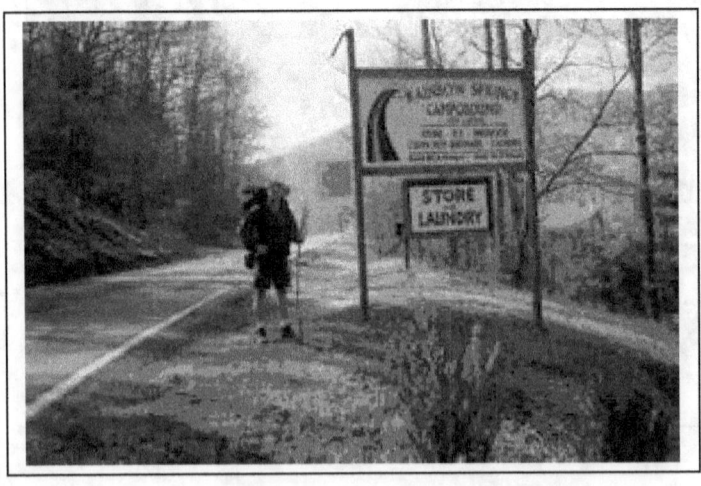

This was just an incredibly beautiful area, and right on the Nantahala River. I was so captivated with this campground that several years later, Terry and I spent two months camping there. In that utopian spot and with the perk of extremely reasonable fees, just $10.00 per day which included all utilities, it was my idea of what heaven might be like. Ultimately, we became good friends with the campground's owners. It was sometime during these years that Bill Bryson's book arrived upon the scene, shedding a less-than-stellar light upon this campground, actually relating to 'the deplorable conditions' of the bunkhouse. Fearing a backlash from the negative publicity, the owners decided to put the property on the market. Sadly for Rainbow Springs, it was purchased by a large Atlanta real estate conglomerate, whose intent was to turn those glorious 10 acres into sites for million dollar homes. However, the process of obtaining all the necessary permits, and courting the politicians of Macon County, in order to enable a development of such tremendous proportions took time, even for the big guys. (This was, after all, abutting the Appalachian Trail, not your typical residential acreage). Consequently, the campground stayed open and fully functional for two more years while all the issues and obstacles to the proposed development were wrestled with and hammered out. Though, while open and operating, the developers still needed some on-site management.

The now former-owners suggested that Terry and I would be an ideal choice for that position. So after being 'vetted' with criminal checks, credit checks, and everything else they felt necessary, we were offered the position. It was a good match for all concerned, and the base salary was a fair one. Terry would run the camp store, oversee all registrations, and operate computer services. I would be the maintenance guy, grounds keeper, lawn mower guy, firewood chopper, building super and social director. It was a good fit for us and a job made in heaven for the next two years.

Here I must explain how important this camp, and its location, was to the Appalachian Trail. Situated just one mile downhill off the Wallace Gap, from its inception it was designed to be a major stopping-point for thru-hikers on their way up to Maine. For a thru-hiker to reach Maine's Mt Katahdin before the snows of October, he or she must begin their trek in mid February, while the snows of late winter still linger in the higher elevations of Georgia and North Carolina. Needless to say, the weather can play havoc with a hiker this early in the season upon mountain trails meandering 5000 to 6000 feet above sea level. Rainbow Springs, therefore, was ideally and strategically located to serve all the needs of these thru-hikers in what were often perilous conditions. Here, at Rainbow Springs, we provided any and all items they might need at the general store, for at this juncture in their trek, their supplies would have run low, or been depleted altogether.

Our little general store made available everything they might need in order to move on. Another huge plus while we managed this camp, we replaced the old bunkhouse (the infamous Bill Bryson one) with a yurt, a far more comfortable accommodation for the overnighters.

We acquired this amazing piece of housing through the generosity of a local business that had been using it as a store-front. In preparation, I built a sturdy wooden platform, and once the yurt was installed upon it we

121

furnished it with thirty bunk beds, a gas heater, and a refrigerator. It was a marvelous addition to the grounds and a very welcome perk for the hikers.

As for the old maligned bunk house? I converted it into a sauna, warmed by a great little wood-fired stove, and with walls lined with sweet-smelling cedar. Trail weary hikers, cold, wet, and weary, absolutely loved it!

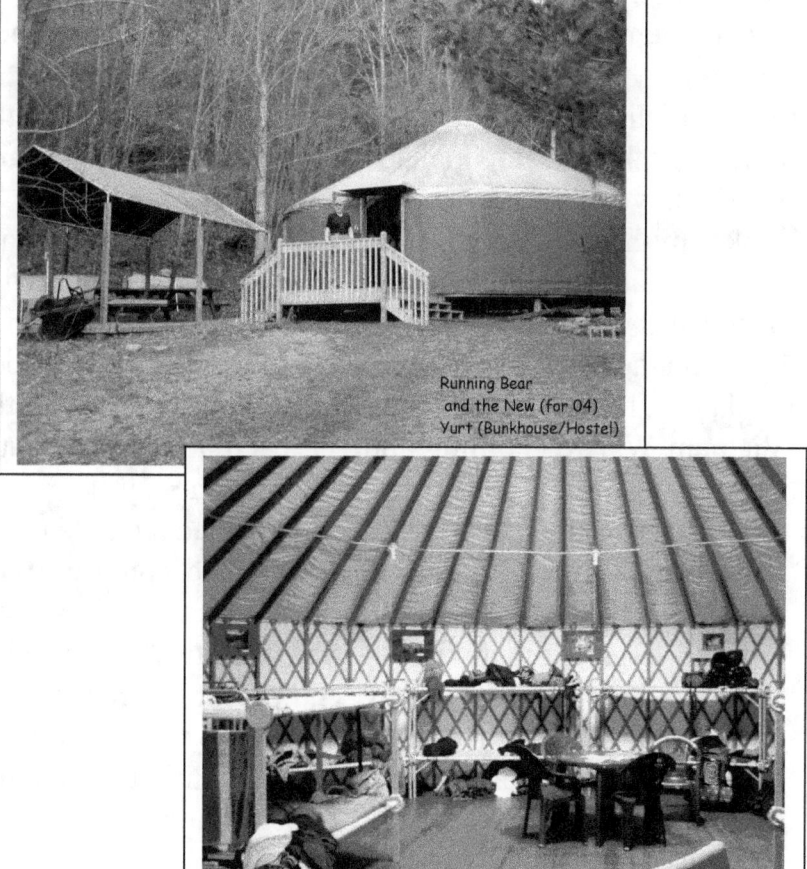

Running Bear and the New (for 04) Yurt (Bunkhouse/Hostel)

Yurt aka Bunkhouse

For some time I'd been giving each hiker a stamped postcard addressed to Rainbow Springs with the instruction to drop them in the mail when they reach the end of their journey at Maine's Mt. Katahdin. They're usually pretty beat up when we receive them back, but it's a kick to get them and read the hikers notes scrawled upon them. It makes me feel that somehow we played a small role in their successes. These postcards were always displayed on the bulletin board right next to the pot bellied stove for all to see. It added a measure of encouragement to those thru-hikers following in their footsteps.

Well, we knew the end was coming and by the third year the developers had all their 'ducks in a row' and were ready to 'out' us, and vanquish the campground. It broke my heart to see this beautiful and vitally important camping facility vanish, to be replaced by urban sprawl. I believed it was not only a crime against the Appalachian Trail, but against nature herself. So Terry and I developed a plan. I hadn't been an anti-war protester during the Vietnam War for nothing and "I'd been a rebel without a cause now for too long." I was ready for the fight!

These big guys from Atlanta dangled a challenge in front of us. They told us that if we could come up with one million dollars they would sell it to us. So, Terry and I began a gargantuan fund-raising effort. We contacted sixty companies that supply equipment to hikers and outdoorsmen: Sierra Designs, L.L. Bean, and North Face to name a few. Then I spent night after night contacting every hiker who had stayed at the campground during these past two years begging their support in any way possible; imploring them to write or call all their friends, all their equipment suppliers, beseeching them to put in a supporting plug for our grant application.

The Appalachian Trail Conference and The Land Trust for the Little Tennessee also became involved and supported our efforts. The major concern of the Land Trust folks was the probable compromising of the river's headwaters, which is just as short stretch from the protected National Forest.

The ground under Rainbow Springs is riddled with springs creating a series of rivulets leading directly down to the pristine Nantahala River. This river is famous as a breeding ground for its famous and magnificent Rainbow trout. It was ludicrous to imagine a development of any sort defiling this unspoiled area. The run-off alone from the development of this land would ruin the now crystal-clear river waters, likely obliterating the riverbed that now sparkles through 4-feet of icy clear water. Additionally, the porous soil of the area might not even support the necessary septic tanks of the proposed home sites. "We simply did not need a bunch of condominiums sitting here on this river."

Alas! All was in vain. One million dollars was a lot of money, and although we had the concerns, and sympathies of hundreds of campers, hikers and outfitters, *plus* their very generous financial contributions, we just couldn't raise the necessary funds. Rainbow Springs was lost. The developers won. All monies were returned to those who supported the heroic effort.

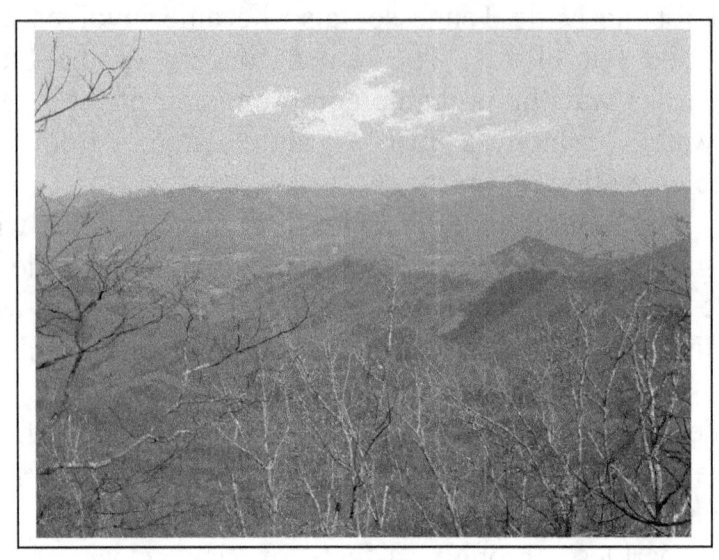

View from Albert Mountain Campsite

Appalachian Trail Terminology

* **Thru-hiker:** A hiker that completes the entire 2,174 miles of the AT in one fell swoop. A thru-hiker takes five months on average. Most start in Georgia in mid-March, after risk of snow has passed and finish in Maine on late August before winter weather hits Mount Katahdin.

* **South Bound:** A thru-hiker is one who starts in Maine and hikes to Georgia. Only an average of 15 percent of all AT hikers are south-bound hikers.

* **Section-hiker:** This applies to those who hike the Trail in sections rather than attempting to complete it in one undertaking. For some this may mean a 20 or 30 year commitment.

* **2,000-miler:** Anyone who completes the entire trail. This can be a thru-hiker or a section hiker.

* **Flip-floppers:** This is a hiker who leaves the trail at one point and picks it up at another.

* **Mail drops:** Hiker often calculate where they will be on a certain date and when they might run out of supplies and self-address care packages to themselves to arrive at the designated spot at the designated time.

* **Zero day:** This term is used by hikers who logged no miles on that day. Possibly resting, doing laundry or escaping bad weather.

* **Triple crown:** A hiker who completes all three major trails in the continental United States: The *Appalachian Trail* at 2,174-miles, the *Pacific Crest* at 2,650, and the *Continental Divide* at 3,100 miles.

* **Trail name:** Many hikers adopt a trail name. It can be a deep and symbolic name or nonsensical one.

* **Trail log:** A notebook maintained at every shelter, campground and hostel on the AT and used to communicate with fellow hikers regarding plans, whereabouts and conditions, or simply to note a silly poem, cartoon, or thoughts for the day.

Chapter *Fifteen*
Rainbow Springs - Part II

In 2005, upon Rainbow Spring's closing, our mission became an all out effort to create and maintain a replacement hostel for the support and comfort of those early spring thru-hikers, especially during the inclement weather they would undoubtedly confront. So, in early March, not unlike Don Quixote and his quest to right all wrongs, we left New Smyrna Beach, Fl. in a 1976 Dodge 22' camper, towing a small Dodge pickup that overflowed with all the necessary provisions to make it happen.

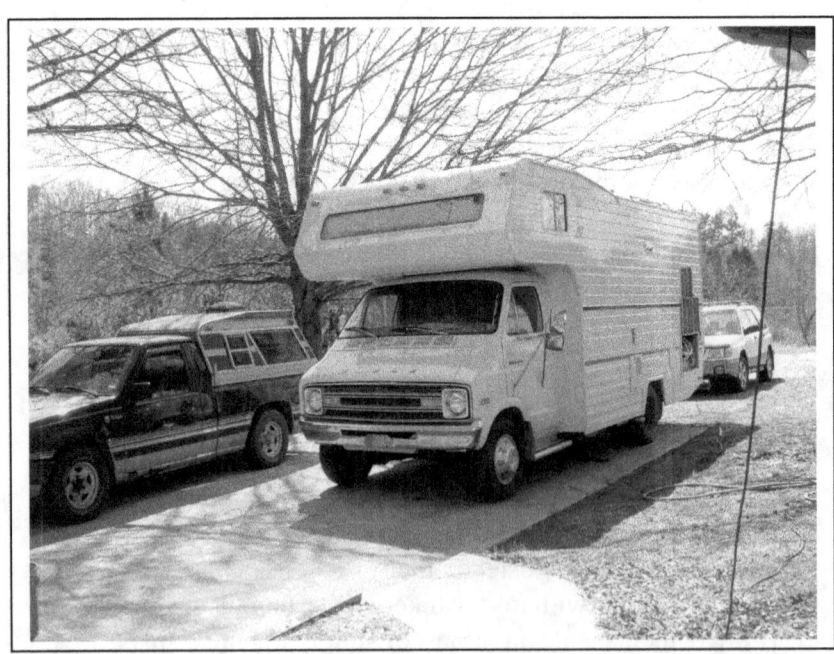

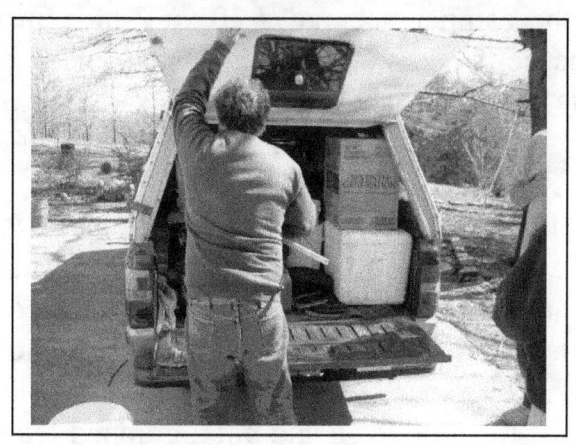

To aid and abet our efforts our friends from Clancy's Cantina in New Smyrna Beach (yes, the same Clancy's that once supplied us with veggie oil fuel), sought the support of their suppliers, who in turn provided food that consisted of 4,000 tortilla shells, 100 lbs. of dried beans, (black and pinto), 50 lbs. of rice, 30 lbs. of shredded Mexican cheese, 2 gallons of jalapeno peppers and 3 cases of #10 cans of chopped tomatoes, (for homemade salsa), and all at wholesale prices. They also gave us their blessings and their coveted recipes for the "Best Ever" roll your own burritos. Then we linked up with Mike, (aka Gator Aide), a friend from Jacksonville, in the western North Carolina Nantahala Forest.

We were granted access to Albert Mountain on March 15, 2005, courtesy of the Forest Service, who, with much effort (it was still winter up there) opened the service gate, and helped us get everything hauled up the mountainside. Time was of the essence as we had to get set up before an impending blizzard was forecast to arrive. We set up at 5,000 feet, near the base of Albert Mountain, and 100 miles from the start of the Appalachian Trail. Racing against the weather, we leveled the camper, secured a 30'x60' tarp, installed the solar electric system which consisted of two 80-watt BP solar panels, a charge controller, plus two 12-volt gel cell batteries, and in the event of extreme weather conditions, a 1,000-watt back up generator.

Once all the necessities were in place, I assembled a "Maine Lumberjack Griddle" from a 75 year old, 36" circular sawmill blade, which I had resurrected from my grandfather's farm in Maine. This was suspended from a tripod of 5/8" rebars with cables to raise or lower it. It became the most beloved and photographed feature of our camp.

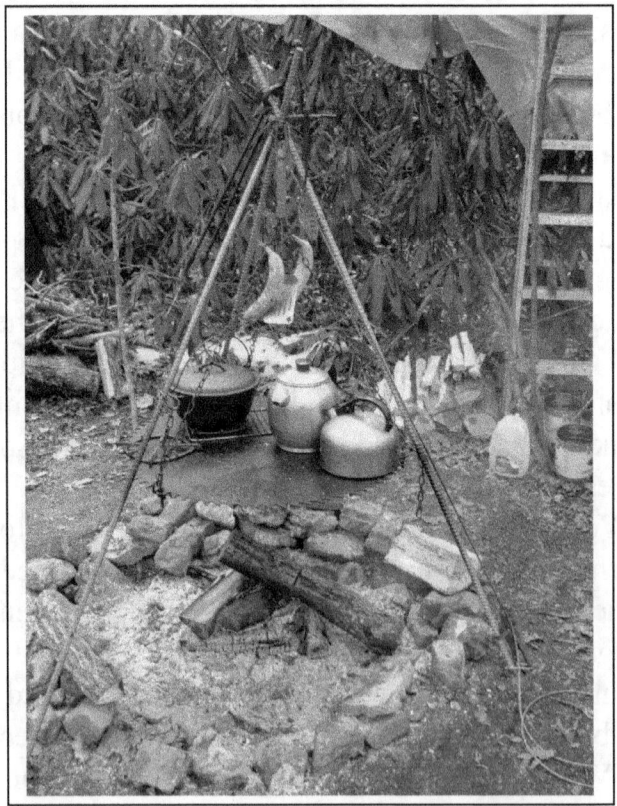

Also included in the initial set up was the construction of a rustic latrine, plus a rain barrel collection unit (for washing, bathing and laundry as the crystal-clear springs nearby would supply our drinking water), the building of a fire pit, crowned with the "Maine Lumberjack Griddle", and the creation of a huge three-room tent for sheltering the hikers. We then tuned in the satellite radio, and finally strung up LED Christmas lights. (Which use less than 1.8 watts per strand). Steve, a former AT thru-hiker, at *Real Goods** helped us obtain a charge controller, bio toilet paper, and a solar sourcebook, (which was to become the "Sears Catalog" of the hiker's latrine).

About that latrine, rather than a whole bunch of 'cat holes' about the camp (these are the shallow holes dug by campers in the wild to deposit their waste, aka: poop and then cover over, just as a cat would), I solved this dilemma by 'manufacturing' a latrine out of a 5-gallon bucket hovering above 4-foot deep hole, a conventional toilet seat, and a tarp for privacy. It served the purpose!

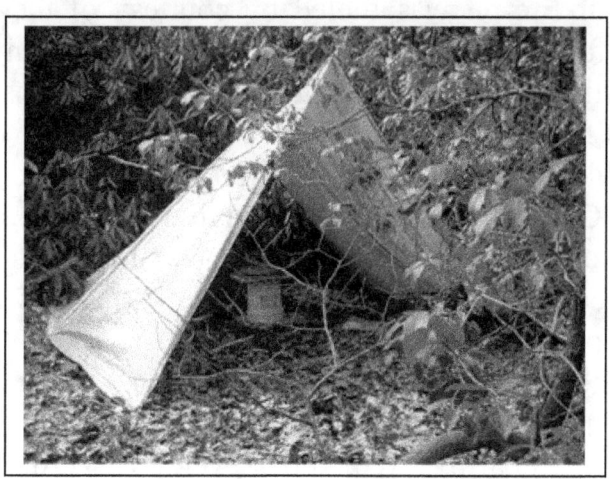

Terry began cooking, and we were ready for hikers! Mission accomplished.

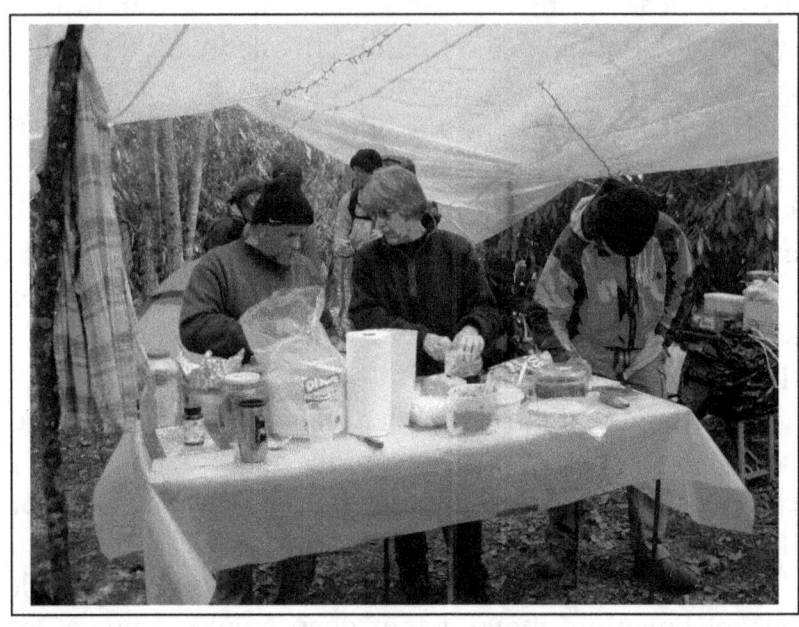

Our fire-pit was fueled by courtesy of the Forest Service folks who granted us permission to cut any dead wood, either fallen or standing, and with our chainsaw we kept this fire going non-stop for 32 days.

Hikers on the trail, cold, wet and dog-tired would see our Christmas lights, hear our music and gratefully fall into our camp. They could eat, warm up, sleep in relative comfort, and rally their bodies and souls for the next leg of their journey.

They would slap a tortilla on the grill and once heated through, would fill it with all the good stuff Terry had been preparing. We kept several cast-iron Dutch ovens in the camper continually full of warm black beans

131

and rice. Terry also provided cheese, salsa, onions, and jalapeño peppers. From all these ingredients, each camper would fill and roll their own burritos. Talk about happy hikers! They thought they'd 'died and gone to heaven!' A hundred miles into the Appalachian Trail, they had stumbled upon an oasis of remarkable proportions! The final tally? During those incredible 32 days, we fed nearly 800 hikers!

It was "Trail Magic" at its finest!

* Real Goods Trading Corporation (commonly referred to as Real Goods) is a retail store and mail order / e-commerce business located in Hopland, California that sells renewable energy systems, homesteading supplies, and other environmentally friendly goods and resources for people interested in living off the grid or with a low environmental impact.

Chapter *Sixteen*

Rainbow Springs - Part III

IT WAS REALLY ALL ABOUT THE PEOPLE

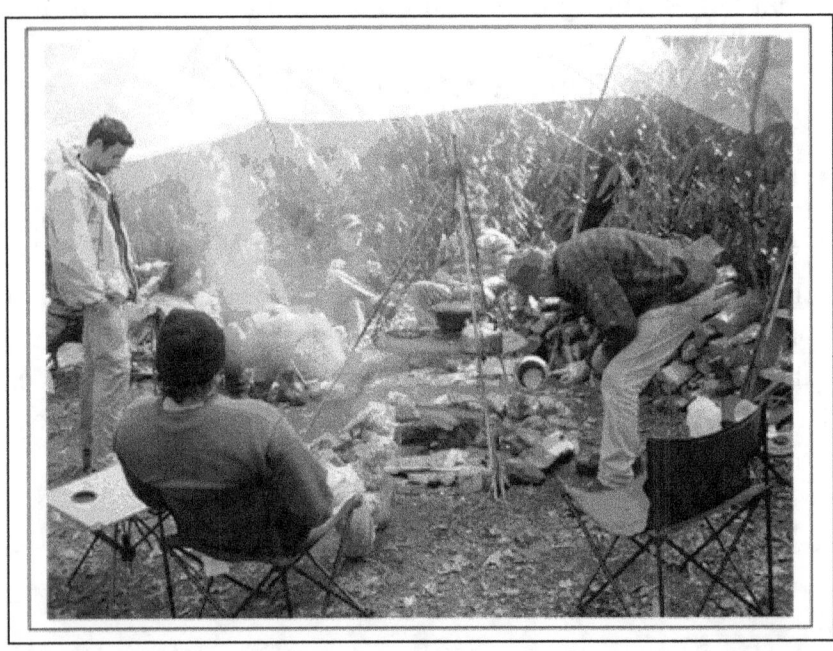

We were thirty two days on the mountain, and the longest, then known, of running "Trail Magic". We supplied nearly 800 thru-hikers with 4,000 burritos, provided over 300 gallons of coffee, cases of soda, shelter, and a hot campfire that never went out, and sometimes breakfast, compliments of Gator Aide and Fishin' Fred.

None of this could have occurred without the people who became our allies in this cause. They are called "Trail Angels". A "Trail Angel" may be described as a generous individual, or a group of individuals, that provide random acts of kindness to other hikers along the trail. This may be in the form of providing food and water, giving medical aid, offering transportation, or simply a friendly encouraging word. Aside from fellow hikers, there are whole communities just off the trail, that are considered "Trail Angels" as well, often leaving fresh water and other necessities within easy reach of a hiker coming down off the trail. All these "Angels" are closely associated with "Trail Magic" and "Trail Magic" might best be described as something unique along the trail; a place or event that has a knack of occurring just when a hiker's spirits are approaching the danger zone. Aka: Rainbow Springs!

Our "Trail Angel" brigade began when two hikers arrived at camp on their way north, and quickly realized that the services we were providing could use some additional assistance. Terry and I had truly bitten off a big chunk and were stretched to the limit. 'Fishin Fred' and 'Gator Aide' (these are trail-names bestowed by fellow-hikers), were the first to see the impact our camp was making, and immediately grasped our need for more hands. They tabled their hiking agenda, rolled up their sleeves, and pitched in for the duration of the stay. 'Fishin Fred' was from Michigan, a tree arborist, and an expert with a chainsaw, and he kept us supplied with firewood. 'Gator Aide' was great in medical emergencies, for he had a 4-wheel drive Chevy and could quickly transport someone down into town for help when the situation required it.

IF WE HADN'T BEEN THERE

Early one morning, probably around 4 am, I got up, and through the glow of the firelight, I saw someone huddled next to the smoldering fire pit. I first thought it was 'Fishin Fred', but when I called out to him, the poor startled fellow jumped nearly out of his skin. He immediately began apologizing, explaining that he had followed our lights into camp. He had fallen off the trail, and was very wet and was badly bruised, plus he had lost all his camping gear in the process. This guy, who we later dubbed as 'Biker Bear', for prior to attempting the Appalachian Trail he had successfully bicycled his way across the country, had begun his hike very poorly equipped. His Wal-Mart sneakers were totally inadequate for trail hiking, and with the traction-less shoes on his feet, he had attempted to negotiate some rather infamously challenging ledges to our south. To traverse these ledges (no wider than a foot and a half) one must cling firmly to the ledge, with face and body pressed tightly against the ledge, while rear-end and backpack dangle precariously out over the edge. 'Biker Bear' had attempted this hazardous crossing at night, and in a freezing rain storm. The results could have been disastrous, for he fell 60 feet into the ravine below. Once he'd gathered his wits, he jettisoned all his gear, and crawled his way back up. He was alive and a bit beaten up, but now in a very serious situation; wet, cold, hurt, no equipment, and no idea where he was. As he began to make his way to 'who knows where' he saw our Christmas lights and campfire off in the distance. He thought he was imagining it, that it was a mirage, and that he had surely lost his mind, but made his way in that direction anyway.

When I discovered him at 4am, he was on the verge of hypothermia. We hustled him into the heated camper, got him out of his wet clothes, bundled him up in warm blankets, and settled him on the couch. Once he recovered and felt strong enough to make a decision, he declared that his hiking days were over, and he wanted to get the heck off this mountain! 'Gator Aide' obliged and drove him down into town. There is no doubt in my mind that we saved his life that night. The nearest place of refuge was 11-miles up the trail, and he would never have made it! Sometime later, a hiker stumbled upon his discarded equipment but 'Biker Bear' was long gone.

Soon after that situation, we were notified by a group of thru-hikers that there was a poorly-equipped girl back on the trail who was in need of some serious intervention. Her choice of footwear (again) had been sneakers, and now her sneakers were nearly worn through, and her feet were raw. 'Fishin Fred' and 'Gator Aide' immediately began hiking back down the trail to find her. She was in such bad shape that she could no longer walk, and the guys had to carry her back up to our camp. When she arrived we had to physically cut her sneakers away from her bloodied and mangled feet. We soaked her feet in warm water, long enough to remove all traces of the sneaker fabric and then doctored her with Merthiolate antiseptic. It stung like the devil, and she screamed in pain. However, it averted any possible infections. When she had recovered enough 'Gator Aide' transported her down off the mountain and (hopefully) to a wiser understanding of what it takes to hike a mountain trail. Sometime later she contacted us to thank us for all we did for her.

~ ~ ~ ~ ~ ~

The Log Book Tells the Whole Story

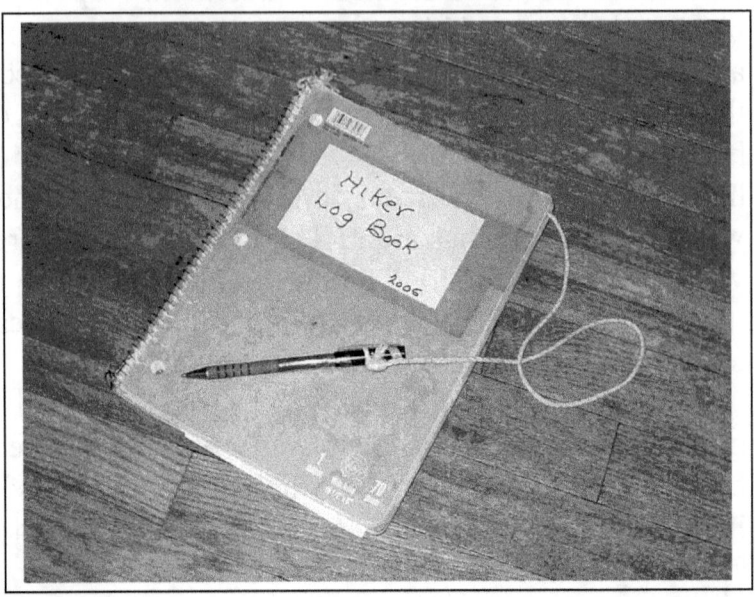

These are just a sampling of the hundreds of comments left behind by the many hikers who stumbled upon our little bit of "Trail Magic."

3/17 - The oasis is one thing, however the loving people who are taking care of us when we need the warmth, food and loving kindness is truly a "God" send. I will miss this wonderful trail magic and can only say "Thank you for what you are bringing to this trail."

Love ~ Forever North and Woody

3/18- The traverse from Mooney Gap left me spellbound with the beauty of this place. Six bean burritos, great kinships, and Jimi Hendrix blarin' on the stereo left me spellbound with the people and their kindness.

Many thanks and blessings ~ Buttah

3/25 - Best Trail Magic ever! The world is full of good folks!
Thank you! ~Tent Shaker

3/26 - Salsa, salsa. salsa, salsa . . . mmmn, mmmn Thanks to Gator-aid, Fishing Fred & Barry for making food dreams come true. I will never dread a hill again. Mmn, mmn, mmn . . . back to beans & rice again.
Hey to all! ~ Gypsy LuLu

3/27 (Easter)- Mrs. Barry, we came in on a cool, slippery, rainy Easter Day, and we were greeted with a fire, a dry place to sit, happy faces, AND your wonderful corn chowder!
Merci! Thank you! and God Bless! Love ~ Calicoe

3/29 - I thought I smelled onions about 2 miles away. I thought it was a nasal mirage. This is an amazing setup making an already wonderful day perfect.
~ Rockin' Steady

3/30 - If this is Trail Magic then you guys are MAGICIANS!
Thanks for the grub! ~ Squeaker

4/1 - HOLY COW! 2 days of rain! Wet tent, clothes, and hiking in the rain up to Albert Mt. "Where is it?" I say. Then came upon a sign that says "Trail Magic" - a total oasis in the woods. Probably the best set up yet, and the best part was the Maine Lumberjack griddle.
Thank you and good luck! ` Lost Baggage

4/2 -I always say the things people miss most on the trail are 1) food, 2) music, 3) sex, and 4) beer. You've provided us with 2 of them! The best experience thus far and perhaps on the entire trail.
Much love & thanks to you! ~ Southpaw & Nipmuk

4/2 - This was amazing! Saints are required to perform 3 miracles. You guys performed more just while I was here!
~ Zeno

4/2 - About as perfect as it can get. As we Maine folks like to say "Supah!"

~ Brian

4/2 - Snowy Days are not too fun, however Southern hospitality, Trail Magic, and warmth rock my world!

~ Moonpie

4/5 - Trail Magic rumors for two days. Thanks for not being a 'vicious' rumor.

Thank guys ~ Coyote

4/5 - Trail Magic and PEACE in the MIDDLE EAST!

~ Firedog

4/7 - On the most miserable of days I finally got some real food!

Thanks Trail Magic ~ Sasquatch

4/7 - Forget Waffle House. These pancakes were AWESOME!

You made my day! ~ Bluefox

4/8 - I came in the back door, raided the kitchen, and will leave thru the front. Thanks for the burrito, pop, and coffee.

~Hushpuppy

4/8 - They call it "Trail Magic" for a reason for out here it is truly magical!

You guys rock! ~ Sunflower

4/9 - Nice Maine grill. I'm a Mainer myself.

Thanks a billion . . . ~ Kelly

4/11 - That is one hell of a set up! Nothing says 'damn good morning' like breakfast off a sawblade & rebar.

Thanks! ~ KingFu

4/11 - This actually is Trail Magic!! Thank you so much for your heartfelt treatment.

139

~ Jack-a-roo (Whistling Jackrabbit) from Japan

4/12 - Wet and cold! Man this is GREAT!

~ Stump

4/13 - Holy Macaroni! This is INCREDIBLE!

~ Joe

4/13 - I stayed at Rainbow Springs last year. Sorry to hear it has closed. Thank you guys so much for filling in the gap.

~ Icebreak

4/15 - Great 'accidental' stop. Much thanks.

~ Roadie

4/16 - Simply, thank you!
~ from Stopalot and Flying Dizzy from Alaska

4/16 - You guys set the standard and it's F#g!'N high!
Thanks a lot! ~ Nate

4/16 - You guys added another page to my memory album.
Thanks so much ~ Low Gear

4/16 - Last Day of a Great Thing! Barry, Terry, and Gator Aide, what a pleasure and honor to be a part of this with you all. Thanks Much!
Coo Coo Ka Choo! ~ Fishin Fred

4/16 - The last day of a wonderful month plus. Barry, Terry, Fishin Fred, Sam, Ann, and Keith, what a pleasure and fun time we've had. Thanks for all the good times and the friendship.
Happy Trails ~ Gator Aide

The reality of this herculean effort is legendary. There are songs written about the relationship of Terry and I to this all-important campground/hostel, plus videos, reams of notes, letters, and thank you's compiled in the campers' logs - lovingly preserved, and documenting those extraordinary 32 days on the mountain.

And how does this all relate to Chaga Hunting? It was from my experiences on the Appalachian Trail that I came to be hired by the Appalachian Mountain Club of New England for the job in Maine - *and that is what led me to the discovery of Chaga.*

Chapter *Seventeen*

Caveat Emptor

BUYER BEWARE!

Cultivated Chaga? You bought *cultivated Chaga?*
NOOOOOOOOooooooooooo$_{ooooooo}$ · · · ·
Let me share with you the unvarnished truths about cultivated Chaga, and what those who manufacture it don't necessarily want you to know.

Some time ago I attended a Fungi Festival (yes, there are such things, in fact there are many scattered about the country), and this particular Festival was being held in Interlachen, Florida, just north of the Ocala National Forest. While Terry and I set up our booth, we had an opportunity to visit the scores of other venders, and chat with the many purveyors promoting their own natural health products derived directly from nature's bountiful mushrooms.

The promoters of this Fungi Festival were proud and excited to be offering a guest speaker reputedly from the largest medicinal mushroom company in the world, and one of their top representatives would be presenting informational seminars throughout the event.

Before the day was over I would have an opportunity to meet with this rep and hear his story in depth about the 'cultivated' Chaga his company produced and promoted. My curiosity about this product was immediately aroused and my inner antenna instantly went into its 'on guard' mode. "How can something that requires years to grow on a birch tree, deriving its potency and health-giving properties directly from its host, be 'cultivated'," I thought. Well, I was to soon discover the dirty little secret.

A little background first: The future of wild Chaga is in jeopardy. Its use has become so popular, especially in the northern hemispheres, that it is in danger of being overharvested. This is particularly true when novice Chaga hunters improperly hack the Chaga from its host tree. In Russia the government has created a systematic approach to prevent overharvesting. However, in this country, where wild goldenseal, indigenous echinacea, and ginseng are essentially gone, it is feared that wild Chaga will become the next victim of blatant overharvesting. Highly-motivated commercial foragers are rapidly harvesting the more easy-to-access Chaga readily found along the edges of the more accessible back roads and hiking trails. I felt strongly, along with many of my fellow Chaga Hunters, that this careless rape of one of nature's most valued gifts is of extreme significance, and that it is of great importance for our Forestry ecologists to acquire an understanding of this issue and take steps in protecting this valuable asset.

Now more about cultivated Chaga: Research indicates significant differences in the composition between extracts based on wild-harvested Chaga and those based on cultivated Chaga. The sterol composition and the phenolic compounds are completely different. The therapeutic effect of these cultivated compounds is also much lower, or totally absent. In addition, cultivated Chaga contains none of the essential polyphenois, such as melanins, which occur naturally in the Chaga when its host tree is dealing with the harsh habitat in which it grows. Active ingredients such as betulin and betulinic acid are also missing.

That said - back to the eager entrepreneurs who are scrambling, ineffectively, to capitalize on this looming void.

The guest speaker was supposedly a 'big-wig' with the company (the company shall remain name-less for now) and was reputed to boast an impressive scientific background. He apparently was the 'front man' for the company, presenting these informational seminars all over the country. Before the end of the event, following his slick, polished presentation he wandered over to my booth, and with apparent great interest in my Chaga products began to quiz me about it. He, in fact, purchased a significant amount of my product, as he bragged to me about his company being the largest producer of cultivated Chaga in the country. *My antenna was resonating at warp speed.*

As I plied him with questions I immediately began to realize that *beyond a doubt* 'cultivated' Chaga was not only a poor imitation of the real thing, but a totally deceitful product as well. Here's the story:

This company is based in Nevada and so my first question related to obtaining the Chaga. "Do you have it shipped in to you? It must be kinda pricey to have Chaga shipped all the way to Nevada" I queried. He explained that they maintain HUGE warehouses, covering many acres of land, and these warehouses overflow with wood chips, which are inoculated with Chaga spores, and allowed to cultivate, and grow something akin to Chaga. These are NOT BIRCH WOODCHIPS - but any kind of wood chips they can readily obtain.

My mouth dropped open and I stammered, "If you know anything about Chaga, and you certainly claim to, then you must realize that Chaga can only grow on a birch tree. It is from the birch that it derives its life-giving attributes."

He agreed that this was so, but countered with the explanation that 'technically' Chaga will grow on other trees as well. When I continued to quiz him further he stated that they obtained some quantity of wild Chaga shipped in from Michigan and with this they create a 'blend' of the phony (my word) Chaga, combined with a token amount of the true wild Chaga. "So," he continued, "the capsules we produce are a 50/50 blend of both and therefore we are allowed, by law, to advertise it as a 100% Chaga product. It's an advertising ploy."

Deceitful? Hell YES! And his final volley?... after studying the many pictures I display at my booth of recent Chaga harvests, he offered to buy me out! I was so incensed and disgusted that I could barely look at him.

And *that*, Dear Reader is what you must beware of if you purchase Chaga online, or even at your local health-food market. Know who you are buying this from. A true Chaga Hunter who markets only that which he or she harvests himself, can truly attest to its known ability to promote and support your good health and wellbeing.

Chapter Eighteen

NOW FROM THE DISTAFF SIDE

If you are fortunate enough to wander into a farmer's market, street fair, or other neighborhood event at which Barry is marketing his Chaga products, and you let your eyes wander a bit to the right of his spread, you will discover that abutting his display, is an exhibit of lovely and unique beaded jewelry. No surprise that these pieces are crafted by his wife, Terry, and also it should be no surprise that, as they share space with the healing products of Chaga, these handsome bobbles are also designed to aid and abet the wearer in surprising ways.

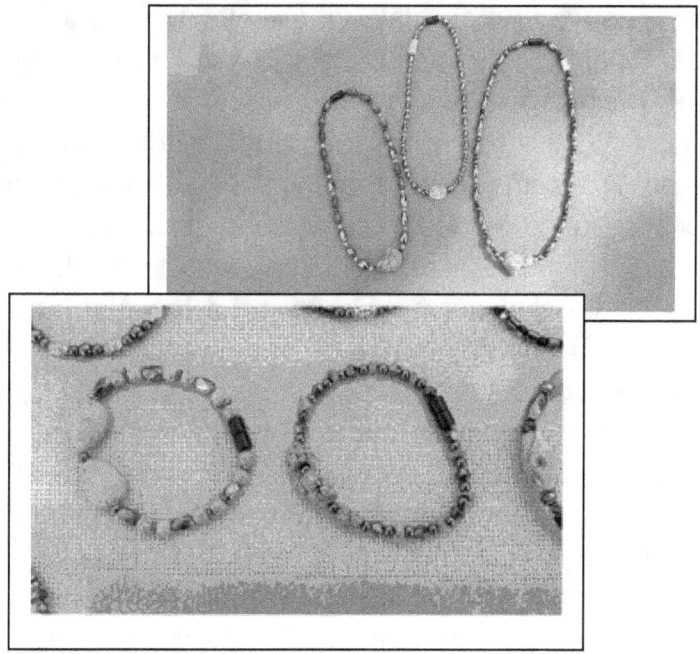

What make these attractive jewelry pieces so exceptional are the curious little black beads that are strung intermittently among the bright, colorful, and vibrant stones and the beads that comprise each piece. Those unassuming little black bobbles are magnetite (see more about these at end of this chapter), a naturally occurring mineral that Terry discovered during the year she and Barry first stayed at the Rainbow Springs Campground. The campground owner of this Appalachian Eden had obtained several free passes to the annual Gem Show, now exhibiting just off the trail in the nearby town. Never having been to one before, she and Barry grabbed at the chance to go. At this initial exposure they became enthralled by the vast array of gems, and all the marvelous items that the artisans and crafters were creating from them. They spent hours there, and then returned for several more days of the event! One artist in particular caught Terry's interest. She was crafting beautiful pieces of jewelry; necklaces, bracelets, and pendants, from a stone totally unfamiliar to Terry. The vibrant beaded gems were interspersed with contrasting black beads (magnetite), the properties and potentials of those humble stones amazed her. Terry was 'hooked.' The artist kindly showed her how to string a bracelet, adjust the length to fit any size wrist, tie it off, and finish it up with magnetized clasps for ease of taking it off and on. Those magnetized clasps were a feature on every one of the necklaces and pendants, making them super easy to put on. (Every woman knows what a pain it can be to blindly attempt connecting tiny clasps and hooks at the back of her neck). Before the show was over Terry had purchased a sufficient amount of beads and supplies to create her own designs, and these first creations she gave away as gifts to friends. This little hobby soon evolved into a small business, and she began to market them along side Barry's Chaga.

But it wasn't simply the aesthetic appeal of these pretty little pieces that inspired Terry to launch her fledgling jewelry business. It was those little black magnetized beads, the magnetite (a natural stone) whose properties seemed far more significant to her then simple eye appeal, which prompted her to promote her jewelry. Terry felt - and rightly so - that there was a market out there for these pieces, based upon their therapeutic potential.

Proponents of Magnetic Therapy have a strong following, and although scientific evidence has not yet caught up with the theories of those who support it, there are many, many believers eager to share their case histories. The believers claim that the magnetite increases the circulation of blood throughout the body, activating the iron particles in the human blood stream, thus promoting healing of the affected parts and alleviating pain. Since scientific support relevant to these claims is so limited, it's difficult to determine exactly how magnetic therapy promotes healing, however, proponents maintain that the use of the magnets not only stimulates circulation but relaxes the blood vessels, thereby increasing endorphin levels, reducing muscle tension, and normalizing metabolic functioning.

THE PROS AND CONS

Cancer

Even though claims that magnetic therapy can treat diseases like cancer and multiple sclerosis are unfounded, there is some evidence that it may help relieve the pain associated with these chronic conditions.

Arthritis

In a 2004 study of 194 adults with osteoarthritis of the hip or knee, researchers found that those who wore magnetic bracelets for 12 weeks had a decrease in arthritis-associated pain. Meanwhile, a 2001 study of 64 people with rheumatoid arthritis of the knee showed that 68% of those who used magnetic therapy reported feeling *much* better after just one week.

Chronic Pelvic Pain

In a 2002 study of 32 women with chronic pelvic pain, one group of patients had placebo magnets applied to their abdomens for 24 hours a day while the second group had active magnets applied for the same time period. After four weeks of continuous use, those who received the active magnets reported significantly lower pain levels than at the start of the study.

Fibromyalgia

After six weeks of sleeping on magnetized mattress pads, 12 women with fibromyalgia reported significantly less pain, sleep disturbance, fatigue, and next-day tiredness.

Meanwhile a control group of 12 women, who slept on non-magnetized mattresses, experienced negligible improvements in pain, sleep, fatigue, and tiredness.

More Science on Magnetic Therapy

There is also evidence that magnetic therapy may help reduce neck pain, post-polio pain, and diabetic foot pain. However, in studies of the use of magnetic therapy for relief of chronic low back pain and wrist pain related to carpal tunnel syndrome, researchers found magnets no more effective than placebo treatments.

Research into the benefits of Magnetic Therapy show promise in the treatment of female urinary incontinence, such as shown in a 2004 study of 24 patients, where 58% of participants showed improvement after eight weeks of receiving twice-weekly magnetic stimulation of the pelvic floor.
In some cases, magnets are applied to illness-affected areas with the help of wraps, shoe inserts, self-adhesive strips, belts, *or magnetic jewelry like bracelets, necklaces, and earrings*. Other products include magnetic mattress pads and blankets, as well as magnetic-field-generating machines and even magnet-conditioned water.

~~~~~~

Since scientific support for its use is sadly limited, it's difficult to determine how magnetic therapy promotes healing. However, proponents maintain that the magnets have made a significant difference in their wellbeing: stimulating circulation, relaxing blood vessels, increasing endorphin levels, reducing muscle tension, and normalizing metabolic functioning.

THE BOTTOM LINE

If it works for you, you will be a believer. If it does not work for you, you will of course discount its capabilities as so much voodoo. Terry herself wears a bracelet created with magnetite beads and it works for her. She was experiencing near constant pain in her left arm, a residual holdover from an old injury; however, when she wears her magnetite bracelet the pain subsides to a minimal and tolerable discomfort. As for her sales pitch, she tells her customers that these are pretty pieces to wear, show off, and enjoy, with a possible added perk: a potentially added benefit. She does not tout it as being a therapeutic cure-all, but if it becomes so, the customer is the winner.

CAVEATS

If you're undergoing magnetic resonance imaging (MRI), it's important to avoid the use of magnetic devices. Pregnant women and people with cardiac pacemakers should also forego magnetic therapy.
Additionally, it's important to consult your doctor about the condition you're seeking to alleviate through magnetic therapy and to discuss the potential risks and benefits of magnetic therapy. Self-treating and the avoidance, or delaying of standard care could have serious consequences.

~ ~ ~

Terry acquires her magnetite beads via the internet and she relates the interesting tale of their discovery in that far northern Alaskan wilderness. It seems that during the gold rush days the prospectors and miners who were panning for gold in one particular area had issue with the steel nails popping out from the souls of their boots. Further investigation indicated that the very rocks they were walking upon seemed to be pulling those stout steel spikes right out of their tough leather soles and hardy strappings. Can you imagine the frustration those miners must have felt, with so little means available to them, now to have their boots falling apart? However, those savvy prospectors soon recognized that in those magnetized rocks lay an additional source of income. If they couldn't realize their fortunes in gold, they figured it could certainly be augmented by mining this strange new rock with its bizarre drawing ability. And, thus, a new industry was born.

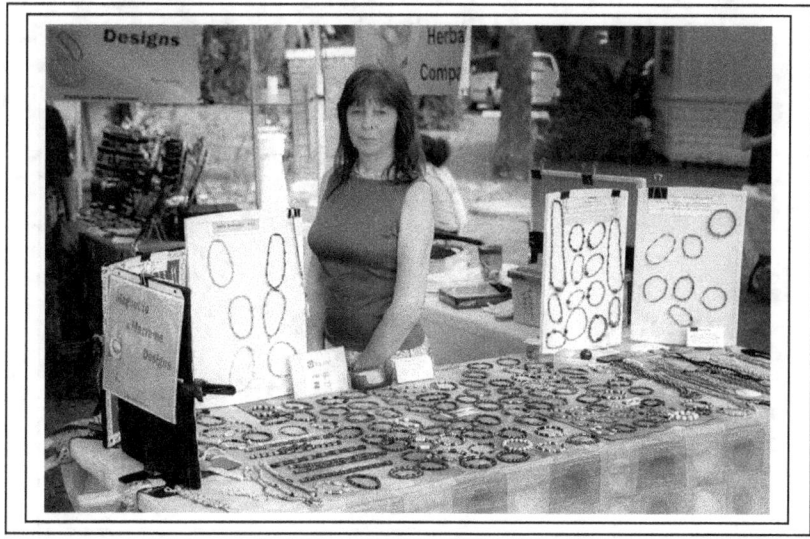

A FEW FACTS ABOUT MAGNETITE

Magnetite is a mineral and one of the three common naturally-occurring oxides of iron. Its chemical formula is Fe_3O_4, and it is a member of the spinel group. Magnetite is ferrimagnetic; it is attracted to a magnet and can be magnetized to become a permanent magnet itself. It is the most magnetic of all the naturally-occurring minerals on Earth. Naturally-magnetized pieces of magnetite, called lodestone, will attract small pieces of iron, which is how ancient peoples first discovered the property of magnetism. Magnetite is best known for its property of being strongly attracted to magnets. Some forms of Magnetite from specific localities are in fact themselves magnets. Commonly known as Lodestone, this magnetic form of Magnetite is the only mineral that is a natural magnet. Due to the magnetism of Lodestone, small iron particles are often found clinging to its surfaces.
Magnetite is sometimes found in large quantities in beach sand. Such black sands (mineral sands or iron sands) are found in various places, such as California, Alaska, and the west coast of the North Island of New Zealand. The magnetite is carried to the beach via rivers from erosion and is concentrated via wave action and currents.

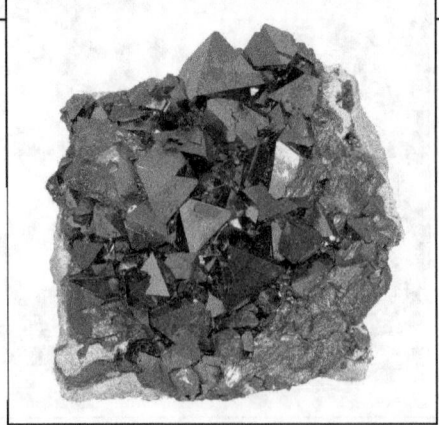

Magnetite as it appears in the rough.

Chapter *Nineteen*

NOW FOR THE REAL STORIES

My name is Dawn and I'm a "Hospice Survivor."

"Terry and Barry, I fully attribute my survival to your Golden Chaga Full Spectrum Tincture.
First, a little about my disease:
I have a quite rare condition called "ossifying fibroma of the mandible." To explain it in layman's terms, I had a benign, but very invasive, tumor that encompassed my entire lower jaw. There was a very thin layer of healthy bone beneath the tumor, holding my lower jaw together. The rest was all tumor . . . fragile, and breakable. To explain - if I got hit in the face (as in a car accident) my entire lower jaw would shatter. In 2015 a "hole" opened up in my jaw and there was a piece of necrotic (dead) bone rattling around in that hole. This made me so very ill (unable to eat, vomiting daily, loosing 25 lbs, terribly weak) that I was placed into the Home Hospice Program and told I had 6 months, or less, to live. At that point I began filling the hole in my jaw with Golden Chaga Tincture twice daily. After one year of daily use, now having been "recertified" by Hospice for another 6 months, a piece of the bone loosened and I pulled it out. It came out in one piece with no bleeding and quickly left a healed, smooth hole in my jaw. I immediately began to get better, and was removed from the Home Hospice Program in March of 2016 for being "too well." I was

cautioned that I now, in all likelihood, had one or more years to live.

Well, live I did! I keep the "hole" very clean, to prevent infection, while still using the <u>Golden Chaga Tincture</u> daily (now under my tongue). Additionally I'm reaping the many benefits of this amazing product. My hair - once so thin that you could see through to my scalp - is growing in and thicker every day.

But - the best gift of all? - I'm convinced that I will live far longer then "they" have predicted for me. I'm painting, driving, walking my dogs, practicing Yoga, dancing, singing, playing my guitar, and gaining back much of the weight I lost. I no longer look like a walking skeleton. When I run into people, who haven't seen me since being admitted into the Home Hospice Program, they are amazed at how well I look.
(They all thought I'd died)

I truly believe that <u>Golden Chaga Full Spectrum Tincture</u> saved my life, and I'm so grateful to Terry and Barry for creating this wonderful product, and making it available to folks in my dire situation! I simply wouldn't be alive without it. I will continue to use it daily for the rest of my life. Not many folks are "kicked out of" Hospice services and I'm sure I wouldn't have been if not for your remarkable gift.

The doctors still label me "terminally ill," but I certainly don't feel "terminal." I'm feeling great! And honestly - aren't we are all "terminal." That's the very nature of our life cycle.

Terry and Barry - Thank you for keeping me alive!"
With much love and gratitude, Dawn Ray

155

READ DENNIS'S STORY

Dennis is a fellow vendor in a nearby booth at one of our venues. For months he'd been listening to me relate the story of Chaga to all my customers and hearing about the many benefits that could be derived from its use. Although he felt he was pretty healthy, he decided to give the tincture a try.

After about eight months of regular use of the tincture he stopped by our booth one day to share his story with us. He and his family have a long history of colon cancer, and he had just recently lost his sister because of it. Because of this condition he has colonoscopies on a very regular basis. He went on to relate that normally the doctor finds many, many polyps and because these can become pre-cancerous it is imperative that they be removed at each procedure. He excitedly told us that at his last procedure the doctor found only one! He attributes this to his daily use of Chaga as he has changed nothing else in his normal routine.   ~ Dennis Hartley

ROB - ANOTHER VENDOR

Just because of the proximity of our booth, Rob couldn't help but overhear me chatting about the benefits of Chaga to anyone who stopped by and showed an interest. Though Rob felt fine, except his walking any distance seemed a bit curtailed, he decided to give Chaga a try. Within a rather short space of time he found that his ease of walking had improved and he was strolling about the marketplace venturing farther and farther each time.

NOW FOR JACK'S STORY

Jack, a rather small, biker guy, his wife, sister, and brother-in-law stopped by our booth several years ago. They seemed quite interested in our Chaga products and listened carefully to all I had to say about the various benefits they afforded. Jack purchased a bottle of *the Golden Chaga Full Spectrum Tincture* and they went on their way.

Just a mere three weeks later, as we were setting up our booth, I glanced up to see Jack, and family, storming across the parking lot heading in our direction. Terry and I glanced at each other both thinking that this is not looking good and we braced for the worst. Jack got to the booth first, slammed both fists down on it, leaned over (we thought somewhat menacingly) and barked, "How much of this stuff can I take!"

Surprised, and a bit taken aback, I answered, "As much as you want."

"Then how much can I buy?" Jack retorted.

I then realized that we weren't in trouble at all, that Jack apparently really liked this stuff and wanted more.

Jack didn't buy out the store, but nevertheless put a sizeable dent in it, and once the business was concluded he quietly confided to me that he had suffered from IBS (Irritable Bowel Syndrome) for many, many years. Not only is this an 'irritating' condition but rather embarrassing as well. With a sideways wink and a smile he related to Barry that in the three weeks he had been using the tincture his condition had improved remarkably. (Another happy customer)

Jack has since been diagnosed with CLL (chronic lymphocytic leukemia). He's been utilizing a lot of Chaga; both the tincture and the tea. Just recently, he reported that the tincture has begun to burn his mouth a bit so he began to cut back on that but still uses the ground Chaga in capsules, and is still drinking tea. I suggested he put the tincture in the tea so he'll still get the full spectrum of the chaga.

His wife related that a normal WBC count ranges from 4500 to 10,000.   Jack's count had been fluctuating between 140,000 and 157,000 and he was getting blood work done every month. Now they have changed that to every 2 months. *"I take that as a good sign."* she said.

ROBERT'S TALE ~ A VIET NAM VET

While in Viet Nam Bob contracted a bacterial infection (nicknamed 'jungle rot'), that 'followed him home' and plagues him all these many years later. Over time countless doctors had offered him a variety of "remedies". Some gave him relief, some didn't work at all. None of them cured it. Bob spent considerable time at our booth, listening with great interest to all I had to tell him about Chaga, and he left with a Chaga purchase.

Just a few weeks later he appeared again at our booth, beaming all over and remarking about the relief he had received from using the Chaga. He is now a regular customer, and user, of three of our Chaga products: the tincture, soap, and the lotion. Here's his story:

"I am a disabled Viet Nam veteran and have struggled with several health issues over the years. I started using a few drops of Chaga under my tongue daily about 1 1/2 years ago. At that time, I had not been able to control my cholesterol numbers or my triglyceride count and had an extreme lack of energy. I was taking long naps and was unable to have a normal life. After using Chaga, my cholesterol and triglyceride numbers have been perfect with every blood test I've had. I no longer have issues with my sugar. I don't need to take those long naps every day and have much more energy. I'm actually back to taking morning walks on the beach with my wife and working in my yard.

I also have been using the Chaga lotion and soap. These have helped suppress my rash that I have not been able to control since Nam. A friend of mine had a severe rash on his back. Several doctors had not been able to help him. I gave him the Chaga lotion and within three days his rash had disappeared.

My wife and I are firm believers in the benefits of Chaga and will continue to use this wonderful product."

~ Robert Kettleband

MEET OLLIE AND HAZEL

This fun couple spotted us at the Eustis Market and stopped to visit. They were from Maine, and as we are too, we chatted long and hard about all the places in Maine that we knew and loved. They also knew a bit about Chaga and had been drinking Chaga tea for quite some time. It was obvious that they walked with some difficulty. It seemed a great effort for them. I counseled them about the value of adding the tincture to their daily routine, as the nutrient rich tincture would offer more healing than the water-based tea. They decided to give it a try with the promise to get back to us with the results.

Just three weeks later they visited our booth again and were obviously walking with greater ease and comfort. They were delighted with their new-found feelings of good health and energy and overjoyed with the long walks they were now able to embark upon.

Ollie and Hazel's story:

"Ollie has always been skeptical about any all-natural remedies, but after hearing about Chaga from a few people, and how it helped them, he thought he would give it a try. Ollie has COPD (chronic obstructive pulmonary disease) and was on oxygen, three inhalers and doing nebulizer treatments 3 or 4 times a day. When he first tried the chaga tea he was only able to walk 100 ft or less without needing to stop a couple of times to catch his breath. After drinking Chaga tea for a few weeks, he was able to walk a lot further. Then he began using the tincture and now he walks around the park and the flea markets without any problem. He has stopped using his oxygen, is down to 1 inhaler and only needs his nebulizer when the humidity is bad. When he went for his annual check-up, his doctor asked him if while in Florida his meds had changed, as his lungs sounded clearer than they had in years. Ollie told him he had been taking Chaga. The doctor said "that can't be it." Ollie insisted that the Chaga gave him more energy so he could walk more. The doctor seemed mystified but we know that it was the Chaga that made this difference!

Then I started taking the Chaga as I was having trouble with walking due to an inflammation in my legs from past surgeries. Now those problems are a thing of the past. When my sister came to visit me from Montana she was having major pain from inflammation in her foot and ankle due to surgeries. At my suggestion she began taking Chaga and it immediately began alleviating her pain. Later, when she went on vacation for a week she forgot to bring her Chaga and by the week's end she couldn't walk without pain. She couldn't wait to get back home and start her Chaga again. Another Chaga success in my family relates to my daughter, Tina. She has suffered a lot of pain due to accidents and her joints really bothered her. She started on Chaga and the pain lessened considerably. Now she would not be without her Chaga."

~ Ollie and Hazel Dalton

MY TURN

A lady never tells her age but I'll share with you that I'm a bit 'long in the tooth'. Now having revealed that fact, you know it's only a short hop to the pharmacy to fill the various prescriptions prescribed by my primary-care doctor. These are the usual mix for a woman of 'my age.' Pills for over-zealous blood pressure, acid-reflex inhibitors for a lifetime of eating all the foods I loved instead of the foods that were good for me, and the little white pills to speed up a sluggish thyroid - plus a handful of over-the-counter capsules that I throw into to the mix, designated to keep me 'up-and-runnin'.

I've been the keyboard behind Barry's voice now for about nine months, and when we started this project

161

Barry began providing me with all things Chaga: the Balm, the Tincture, the Tea, and advice about how to best benefit from their use.

Three months into the project, and faithfully drinking Chaga tea daily as well as slipping a bit of tincture under my tongue each day, I began to experience an uncharacteristic tiredness. I first suspected it to be related to my slow thyroid. Over time my doctor had been adjusting these thyroid pills until my tests proved we had arrived at the optimum dosage. Now, with the tiredness factor looming again, I requested a new test and lo-and-behold it proved that my thyroid wasn't the culprit. Then I wondered if the problem could be related to a dip in blood pressure, so stopped at a nearby CVS, slide into their blood pressure booth and donned the cuff. WOW. My pressure was low! That was a first! The following week I mentioned this to Barry and he shared with me that his wife had experienced the same thing a few months into her Chaga regiment. She had slowly weaned herself off her blood pressure meds and has been doing just fine without them for a number of years.

So . . . I took a deep breath, cut my BP pills in half, bought a BP cuff for home use, and began recording my daily 1/2 dose vs. BP readings. A few weeks into this project I lowered my dosage again, taking the half dose every other day, and still faithfully recording the results. At this writing I'm taking only 1/4 of my original medication and I suspect by the time you are reading this I will be off it completely.

Recently, I burned my thumb, forefinger and palm on the tray of my toaster oven. Since I make my living at a keyboard and a drawing table, having my fingers burned and useless while I waited for them to heal could present a problem. Then I remembered my Chaga Balm. I immediately slathered a tiny bit on each throbbing digit and the burned spot on my palm. It caused additional pain for just a nanosecond then quickly subsided. I proceeded to monitor the burned areas, checking them every few minutes. Within a half hour the pain had completely subsided and the redness was quickly fading away. One hour later my hand looked as though it had never experienced a burn at all! I was amazed! I only wish I had recorded this astonishing recovery on camera.

~ Margaret Rose Scribner

Fishin' Fred's Story

You remember this guy from my stories about Rainbow Springs and how important he was to our Appalachian Trail Magic. Here's his story about the battle he waged against Lyme's Disease and the role Chaga played in combating it.

This is a very nasty disease. It's a bacterial infection primarily transmitted by Ixodes ticks, also known as deer ticks, and on the West Coast, black-legged ticks. These tiny arachnids are typically found in wooded and grassy areas. Because my friends and I hang out a good deal of the time in wooded and grassy areas we are very vulnerable to Lyme's Disease. These ticks are about the size of a poppy seed, and because they are so tiny and their bite is painless, many people do not even realize they have been bitten. Once a tick has attached, if undisturbed it may feed for several days. The longer it stays attached, the more likely it will transmit the Lyme and other pathogens into your bloodstream. It can affect any organ of the body, including the brain and nervous system, muscles and joints, and the heart. If it is not diagnosed and treated early, the spirochetes can spread and may go into hiding in different parts of the body. Weeks, months or even years later, patients may develop problems with the brain and nervous system, muscles and joints, heart and circulation, digestion, reproductive system, and skin. It is frequently misdiagnosed as the symptoms often mimic other diseases and illnesses.

These symptoms include fatigue, cognitive impairment, joint pain, poor sleep, mood problems, muscle pain, and neurological presentations. It's nothing to be taken lightly[1]. And - yes - I've had it too.

Poor 'ole Fishin' Fred. Somewhere during the year 2005 we both contracted Lyme's Disease. I was on my way north - heading for the woods of Maine and the progression of the disease in my case was very quick. By the time I got to Maine I was in dire straits and ended up in the emergency room of a local hospital. The rash covered my entire body and it looked like I was wearing Joseph's *Coat of Many Colors*. The nurses were just astounded when they took off my clothes and recorded my dilemma with many pictures. I was put on antibiotics and that seemed to take care of the problem. However, each year following that episode I would 'blossom' out again with the telltale rash, and its accompanying systems - until I discovered Chaga. I was just learning about the properties and benefits of this amazing mushroom and began using it daily. I totally cleansed my system of this terrible curse and I have never experienced another outbreak.

Now back home in Michigan, Fred never sought help for it and within a short time it had totally incapacitated him. It progressed to a state that he simply could not get out of bed. When he finally sought out medical intervention he was in really bad shape. In those days there where two schools of thought about Lyme's Disease - those trained and practicing under the CDC (Center of Disease Control) did not at that time recognize Lyme's Disease, as did the doctor's practicing in the East, where is began and proliferated. Unfortunately for Fred, way up there in Michigan, his condition was not properly identified. His situation rapidly became desperate. His skin began sloughing off, and he couldn't go outside in the sunlight. Finally, in desperation, he found, on the internet, a powerful antibiotic prescribed for the treatment of bacterial disease in tropical fish - doxycycline. Through a veterinarian's website he was able to obtain this for himself. It worked - and probably saved his life.

When I heard of Fred's plight I immediately got in touch with him and related my success story using Chaga. As luck would have it, he had a cousin that lived in the north woods of upper Michigan. He knew what Chaga looked like and obtained a good-size piece of it for him. With this Fred began making tea and drinking substantial quantities of it daily. It did the trick! It cured him.

~ Fred Orser

It is said that you never rid your body of this disease - that it stays forever - just waiting for a chance to burst forth. I refute this for I've been tested on several occasions and have been found to be free of it.

~ Barry Glidden

Diana's Story

"I discovered the benefits of chaga when a friend of mine used it to battle his cancer many years ago. I had not considered using it for my shingles until I met Barry of Golden Chaga at a flea market in Deland in 2012. Now I keep my Golden Chaga tincture by my bedside and I use it faithfully. My immune system is stronger and I no longer suffer with the painful outbreaks of shingles. Thank you for a pure and potent product!"

~ Diane Jackman Skolfield
www.DianesDetox.org

~ Now let me introduce Richard ~

Richard is my senior by a few years and for years has been very receptive to alternative health approaches. Obviously it must work for him, for he's in tremendous good shape for a guy of his age. When he first learned about Chaga, he took to it like "a duck takes to water." He was one of my very first customers and has been enthusiastically promoting it ever since. So, in a way, you might say we have established a business "partnership" of sorts. He's been witness to, and believer in, the many miracles that it can accomplish. As a fellow vender (of Avon products), following the same circuits that we do, he frequently serves as my 'stand-in' when I am away, particularly during my annual harvesting quests. Consequently, he has gathered, and retained, a significant amount of followers in the name of Chaga. The stories he relates here are so numerous and profound that for the purposes of this chapter I will attempt to condense them.

His Stories

Roger approached my booth and queried, "I understand that I can buy Barry's Chaga from you while he's away. Is this true?" Of course I said yes, so he then proceeded to tell me how he had suffered from high blood pressure since his teens. "And do you know what my pressure is today? It's 127 over 76." Then he turned to the lady next to him, rolled up his sleeve and said, "Look at this! Just a year ago this arm was covered with skin cancer and now it's all gone!"

He completed his purchased and the lady stepped forward and said, "I'll take a bottle of that."

The very next week that lady returned, bought two more bottles and related this story. "I take care of a 92-year-old neighbor because she cannot open her hands enough to care for herself. I started giving her this tincture and five days later she has full use of her hands again." Ultimately she purchased a sizable quantity of the tincture, vowing to send it to all her relatives.

The following winter some of those relatives from up state New York, here for the season, descended upon my booth, and so excited were they about this product that they begged for a "distributorship." I sent them over to Barry's booth and leaving him to negotiate whatever arrangements were mutually agreeable.

That was my first experience with a customer's testimonial. My second one came from a teller at my local bank. She related that her husband had been fighting liver cancer for four years. I suggested she have him try a bottle of the tincture, and she agreed to have him give it a try (but only after she did a bit of research online). One month later, as I approached her station, she appeared jubilant. "My husband's cancer is GONE! His doctors are stunned!" With that she ordered several more bottles.

Now - a tale that needs to be told but if made known within the medical community it will be emphatically denied. My own personal licensed M.D. confided to me that his mother was dealing with a cancerous growth on her hip that has been resistant to all conventional cures. Over time I had dared to enlighten him about my personal experiences and observations of the healing powers of Chaga. So, I'm guessing that as a last-ditch effort, he ordered a bottle from me. His mom began applying it to the growth and within days it began to shrink, and then shrivel, and then finally disappeared altogether. Upon learning of this, one of his office nurses asked to buy a bottle for her son, who was ailing from an undisclosed issue. She related a short time later that he had bounced back and was well again.

Now, this doctor, unbeknownst to his colleagues, began giving Chaga to his patients who were undergoing chemotherapy and radiation therapy. The results were astounding. Their blood counts, which are normally affected in the negative from these treatments, remained stable and constant.

Witnessing these successes the doctor soon began giving Chaga routinely to many of his patients. It would be unethical to charge them for a return to good health and wellness.

Chaga is a wonderful thing!

[1] The Centers for Disease Control and Prevention estimate that 300,000 people are diagnosed with Lyme disease in the US every year. That's 1.5 times the number of women diagnosed with breast cancer, and six times the number of people diagnosed with HIV/AIDS each year in the US.

The antioxidant power of the Chaga can be compared to *'an anti-rust treatment and a polishing for the entire body and its inner organs.'*

CHAPTER *Twenty*

PULLING BACK THE CURTAIN

1910
The Opening Act

~ The first peek behind the curtain ~

Sometime on or about the year 1910, two of American's consummate and revered business giants, John D. Rockefeller and Andrew Carnegie, conceived of a new and heretofore unexploited business opportunity --- founded upon the premise that there were vast hoards of humanity suffering from an infinite variety of sicknesses and diseases. To these moguls of American Industry this populace represented a new, and heretofore, untapped 'marketplace.'

~ And so the curtain slowly parts . . . ~

"When the money is coming from a source which has a vested interest in the outcome, then the outcome is going to be that which the donor wishes it to be. It was the Flexner Report[1] that ushered in the 'reform of medical education in America' by the Rockefeller Carnegie Foundation."

~ G. Edward Griffin,
Author, Lecturer, Filmmaker

In 1973, Griffin wrote and self-published the book World Without Cancer and released it, as well as a video; its second edition appeared in 1997. In the book and the video, Griffin asserts that cancer is a metabolic disease like a vitamin deficiency facilitated by the insufficient dietary consumption of laetrile. He contends that "eliminating cancer through a nondrug therapy has not been accepted because of the hidden economic and power agendas of those who dominate the medical establishment" and he wrote, "at the very top of the world's economic and political pyramid of power there is a grouping of financial, political, and industrial interests that, by the very nature of their goals, are the natural enemies of the nutritional approaches to health".

***

"In the late 1800's and early 1900's medical schools offered many different studies: homeopathic, naturopathic, eclectic herbal medicines; all were there, there was not just 'one way' to better health. The Rockefeller Carnegie Foundation was interested in establishing a 'one way.' How to do that? They would take hold of the medical educational system and effectively establish a monopoly, basically eliminating all competition in patenting and controlling petrochemical medical education. This was the result of the Flexner Report - a preordained account which reported that these homeopathic and natural-teaching schools were not pushing enough chemical drugs. And who was producing these drugs? - The Rockefeller Carnegie Foundation.

At this time the AMA was taking a close look at these various homeopathic, chiropractic, and natural schools, and began shutting down the largest of them. In this climate The Rockefeller Carnegie Foundation saw this as an opportunity and begin showering millions of

171

dollars upon the schools of their choice - those that taught their students to treat the populace with chemical drugs - manufactured, of course, by them. Oh, and by the way, since we're giving you all this money, would you object to having one of our staff become a member of your Board of Directors? In a short space of time the Boards of those medicals schools were 'loaded' with members who were in effect paid staff affiliates of the donor, the Rockefeller Carnegie Foundation. Once this top-heavy component was in place the curriculum of these schools swung completely around, embracing only the teaching of pharmaceutical drugs. And so it has remained to this day. Coincidentally, those highly funded schools produced the most highly recognized doctors, and by 1925, this shift in teaching put all those who practiced natural, homeopathic, and herbal cures, completely out of business, and over 1500 chiropractors were prosecuted for practicing 'quackery'.[2] The twenty two homeopathic schools that flourished in the early 1920's dwindled down to two by 1923. By 1950 all of these schools had closed. In the end, if a physician did not graduate from a 'Flexner Approved' school then he, or she, could not find a job anywhere. This is why today, M.D.'s know so little about nutrition - if anything, and nothing about natural healing of the body. The medical industry today is so skewed in the direction of pharmaceutical drugs, which can be patented and produce great profits for the producers, that all possible therapies coming from nature have been totally excluded. The end results of this unholy alliance conclude that the medical profession has simply become a 'lapdog' of the pharmaceutical industry, and sadly most of doctors are completely unaware of this fact, nor do they know the history behind it."

172

~ Dr. Darrell Wolfe, Ac. Ph.D.
Lecturer, Author, Detoxification Expert

Dr. Darrell Wolfe directed The North American Institute for the Advancement of Colon Therapy for 15 years and was also the head of one of North America's leading natural cancer treatment and preventative care centers.

***

DEFINING DISEASE AS A MARKETPLACE

"The above premise, (DEFINING DISEASE AS A MARKETPLACE) created by just a handful of people, has built what is now considered the largest investment industry. This industry thrives on the continuation of existing diseases, and its seeming inability to eliminate diseases and cancers. I call this a 'Propaganda War' and perpetrated by those profiteers of the pharmaceutical industry."

~ Dr. Matthias Rath, M.D
Founder of Dr. Rath Research Institute.

Matthias Rath, M.D. is an internationally renowned scientist, physician and health advocate. His scientific discoveries in the areas of heart disease, cancer and other diseases are reshaping medicine. He is the founder of Cellular Medicine, the groundbreaking new health concept that identifies nutritional deficiencies at the cellular level as the root cause of many chronic diseases.

***

The Medical Industry complex now enjoys a gross vested interested of $2.7 trillion a year.

> *The early definition of the term "doctor" denoted an eminent scholar and <u>teacher</u>.*

***

"One of the first duties of a physician is to educate the masses <u>not</u> to take medication."

~ Sir William Osler 1849-1919
"Best known physician at the turn of the century and still renowned as the most influential physician in history."

***

"In Medical School we are only taught to prescribe patented medication - never the natural cures found in nature."   ~ Dr. Jonathan V. Wright, M.D.
Medical Director & Founder
Tahoma Clinic - Washington

Dr. Wright is a leader in the field of complimentary medicine as he combines allopathic medicine with an extensive naturopathic medical program. He applies his medical expertise in diagnosing and discussing acute and chronic diseases. Under the guidance of Dr. Wright, Tahoma Clinic is staffed with medical doctors, naturopathic physicians, a traditional Chinese doctor (acupuncture), as well as   nutritionists and allergists

***

"Doctors are taught in medical school that they don't get paid for educating clients, but for writing prescriptions."
~ Dr. Irvin Sahni, M.D.
-- Surgeon, Scientist & Lecturer

Dr. Sahni graduated from the Baylor College of Medicine in 1996. He works in Seguin, TX and 2 other locations and specializes in Orthopaedic Surgery and Orthopedic Surgery of Spine. Dr. Sahni is affiliated with Christus Santa Rosa Hospital-New Braunfels and Guadalupe Regional Medical Center.

***

"Today the students graduating from medical schools have been 'brainwashed' because of the subsidization of their professors who are being paid by the drug companies."   *~ Dr. Garry F. Gordon, M.D., O.D.*

Dr. Garry F. Gordon, MD, DO, MD (H), is an internationally recognized expert on chelation therapy. He is on the Board of Homeopathic Medical Examiners for Arizona.

~ and the curtain parts a bit farther ~

> All truth passes through 3 stages:
> 1. It is first ridiculed
> 2. It is then violently opposed
> 3. Finally, it is accepted as being self-evident
> ~ Arthur Schopenhauer
> 1788-1860

In 1913 the AMA (American Medical Association) created an internal department; calling it the "Propaganda Department." Its goal was to eliminate 'quackery.' And what did they consider quackery in 1913? This was at a time when blood-letting was the norm, (George Washington died from it), and Dr. Ignaz Semmelweis[3] was considered a quack when he advised doctors to wash their hands, and instruments between surgeries. Moving forward to 2016, doctors that do not practice chemotherapy are considered the quacks.

***

A LITTLE HISTORY OF CHEMOTHERAPY

"In Italy, during WWII, nitrogen mustard gas was dropped, killing many soldiers. Ultimately when post-mortem autopsies were conducted on the victims it was discovered that the killings agent had in fact caused the victims lymphocytes to have 'dropped out.' It was concluded from this observation that because the lymphocytes in patients suffering from leukemia and

176

lymphoma produce too much, that the use of the very agents that killed could and would suppress those lymphocytes. Thus chemotherapy was born. And so the very nitrogen mustard gas used to kill soldiers was first used to treat patients in the 1940's and a derivation of it is still used today."

~ Dr. Sunil Pai, M.D.
Integration Medicine Physician,
Lecturer & Researcher

Dr. Pai graduated from the Ross University, School of Medicine, Roseau, Dominica in 1998. He works in Albuquerque, NM and specializes in Family Medicine and Holistic Medicine.

***

SO JUST WHAT DOES THIS DERIVATION OF THE KILLING *NITROGEN MUSTARD GAS* AGENT HAVE TO DO WITH CANCER AND YOUR BODY?

A recent and ongoing study divulged that 90 % of all doctors, especially oncologists, would not treat themselves, or any member of their family with chemotherapy.

~ Dr. Sunil Pai, M.D.

Why? Chemotherapy bombards the body with the most highly toxic chemicals known to mankind. This approach to the 'war on cancer' not only kills the cancer cells but also renders those neighboring healthy cells dead as well. But of more importance, and, highly significant in the healing of the patient, is the annihilation of those adjacent stem cells[4]. This attack makes the survival of the patient nearly impossible, almost a miracle, and the agents being used to fight cancer are in fact, cancer-causing chemicals. And so it would seem that instead of eliminating cancer we are inducing new cancers.

~ Dr. Aleksandra Niedzwiecki, PH.D

Dr. Aleksandra Niedzwiecki, a Member of the Board of the Dr. Rath Health Foundation, also serves as an Executive Vice President and Vice President of Research at Matthias Rath, Inc. Dr. Niedzwiecki received her Ph.D. in biochemistry from the University of Warsaw, Poland.

ACT III

~ The curtain opens wide ~

"It is estimated that by the year 2020 that half of all cancers in America will have been medically induced by drugs or radiation. So our medical establishment itself will soon become the leading cause of cancer in America. Statics tells us that 42 to 46 percent of cancer patients actually die from cancer. That means that the remaining 54 to 58 percent of cancer patients die from the treatment. Ultimately when the immune system is suppressed -as it is through chemotherapy - the patient suffers liver and kidney failure, pneumonia and sepsis - a life-threatening condition that arises when the body's response to infection injures its own tissues and organs. So WHY is the medical profession treating cancer with a

178

hazardous drug that is not only ineffective but DANGEROUS, with a propensity to cause cancer rather than cure it? The distressing bottom line is - doctors by virtue of their license are required to do so, and if they refuse will suffer adverse consequences even the loss of their license to practice."

~ Dr. Rashid Buttar, D.O.
Author, Lecturer & Speaker

Rashid A. Buttar, DO, is a graduate of the University of Osteopathic Medicine and Health Sciences, College of Medicine and Surgery. He trained in General Surgery and Emergency Medicine and served as Brigade Surgeon and Director of Emergency Medicine while serving in the U.S. Army.

***

"Once I entered into oncology practice in San Francisco I began studying the 5-year survival rates of cancer patients having been treated with chemotherapy. The results were staggering! Only 2.1 percent survived beyond 5 years!" (This gleaned from the 2004 edition of The Journal of Oncology)

~ Dr. James Forsythe, M.D.

Dr. Forsythe is an author, anti-aging physician, and integrative oncologist specializing in the use of human growth hormone to attempt and slow the symptoms of aging. Forsythe is a former associate professor of medicine at the University of Nevada School of Medicine and frequently appears as the featured speaker at conferences of the American Academy of Anti-Aging Medicine International Congress. He founded the Century Wellness Clinic in Reno, Nevada.

"This was a massive study and I interviewed the lead epidemiologist[5] of this study soon after the report can out. He assured me that the situation was becoming bleaker with an anticipated percent of survivors dropping still further.

The first lie the cancer patient hears is: Chemotherapy.

The second lie is: surgery. The sad fact is the tumor has already become metastatic and surgery 'spills it' further. The patient will be told at some point in his treatment that the cancer has 'come back.' The truth is - it never left!"

~ Bob Wright Founder of AACI
(American Anti-Cancer Institute)

Bob Wright is considered an authentic American "cancer whisperer," he teaches patients how to correct the underlying metabolic basis of the disease to elicit their own body's healing response. Wright is the author of the book "Killing Cancer - Not People"

***

"Currently there is in access of $127 million dollars being spent yearly on ineffective cancer treatments, with the bulk of these funds going directly into the Pharmaceutical Industry."

~ Dr. Sunil Pai, M.D.

"The 'real' war on cancer is a 'turf' war aimed at protecting its profits."

~ Dr. Stanislow Burzynski, M.D., PH.D.

Dr. Burzynski, a nationally and internationally recognized physician/investigator, pioneered the use of biologically active peptides for the treatment of cancer.

*****

And just who is the vigilant pit bull guarding the gates of this lucrative behemoth?   - The FDA (The Food and Drug Administration).

*****

[1] The Flexner Report is the most important event in the history of American and Canadian medical education. It was a commentary on the condition of medical education in the early 1900s and gave rise to modern medical education. The report is named for Abraham Flexner (1866-1959) who prepared it.

[2] Here, I can add a personal story. My mother's first husband was Dr. Justin Barber, an early graduate of Palmer Chiropractic College of Davenport, Iowa. He, along with his mother, brother, and brother-in-law (all licensed chiropractors) established practices in Massachusetts, circa 1924. They looked on in fear and apprehension as one by one the 'authorities' sought out, and arrested many of their fellow practitioners. They themselves were able, by the skin of their teeth, to stay

just one step ahead of those on this unholy quest.
~ Margaret Rose Scribner

[3] On the evening of May 15th, 1850, a prickly Hungarian obstetrician named Ignaz Semmelweis stepped up to the podium of the Vienna Medical Society's lecture hall where many of the earliest discoveries in medicine were first announced. And what, exactly, was the doctor's advice to his colleagues on that long ago night? It could be summed up in three little words: wash your hands!

[4]The importance of the stem cell: Stem cells are still quite primitive and live throughout the entire body. They have not 'decided' what they will become; could be brains cells, or heart, or lung cells. Their DNA can be damaged by free radicals or chemotherapy. Once damaged they become 'immortal' producing more and more and more - literally becoming a cancer. Radiation and chemo treatments will have no effect upon them - only killing their 'offspring'. Because of the complex chemical changes surrounding these 'immortal' stem cells, they become stronger and more aggressive, and the patient experiences a full-blown return of the disease usually resulting in death.   ~ Dr. Russell Blaylock, M.D.
Neurosurgeon, Scientist
Editor of the Blaylock Wellness Report

[5] Epidemiology is the study and analysis of the patterns, causes, and effects of health and disease conditions in defined populations. It is the cornerstone of public health, and shapes policy decisions and evidence-based practice by identifying risk factors for disease and targets for preventive healthcare. Epidemiologists help with study design, collection, and statistical analysis of data, amend

interpretation and dissemination of results (including peer review and occasional systematic review). Epidemiology has helped develop methodology used in clinical research, public health studies, and, to a lesser extent, basic research in the biological sciences.

CHAPTER *Twenty one*

AND AGAIN THE CURTAIN SLOWLY CLOSES
LEAVING THE AUDIENCE IN THE DARK

The first thing the Hippocratic Oath says, which most physicians have never read, is "First, do no harm." Just further down in the Hippocratic Oath, is states, "I will not give a poison, a deadly poison."

However, most of the drugs that we give, particularly in oncological care, have a black-box warning, which means that more people often end up in the black box.

I do not believe that your family physician, nor his or her many colleagues, are involved in some sort of conspiracy to make you, and keep you, unhealthy for the sake of their financial gain. These men and women went into the field of medicine because they had the brain-power to do so, and because they had the strength of character to want to aid and assist in the betterment of their fellowman. I do believe however, that behind a barely visible curtain hovers the driving force propelling this medical behemoth: rewarding all who benefit *their* purpose and long-term goals, and ostracizing *all* who honestly practice and promote otherwise. The victim is the poor soul who wishes to benefit and achieve optimum good health through nature, and proven natural remedies. The practitioner who provides these services, which are not "approved" and therefore "outside the standard of care" is <u>severely</u> penalized for providing it.

FOUR YEARS OF RUNNING ON THE
FDA HAMSTER WHEEL

A Tale from Deep Within
the Woods of Northern Maine

"I was first introduced to Chaga by one of my customers, a lady from British Columbia that I sold birch bark to. The year was 2009 and at that time my major source of income was derived from creating and marketing rustic wooden furniture and other natural wood products. This lady emailed me posting a specific question regarding Chaga - which she assumed I knew about as it grows on birch trees - one of my major product sources. My response was 'What the heck is Chaga?' She replied 'Look it up. Here's a link. It's amazing stuff.' I checked out the link she had provided me with and was intrigued by what I found. I then began delving deeper into all the information that could be found about it on the internet. But sadly, in 2009, there was not a whole lot of information about it out there, and it seemed that no one was marketing any of the products that could potentially be derived from it. Oh My Gosh! I've been seeing Chaga all my life and never knew what it was! To me, it was just an ugly growth attached to a birch tree and something to be totally dismissed. With my new-found knowledge I harvested a good size chunk, brought it home, and brewed up a substantial pot of tea. I kinda liked the pleasant woodsy taste and began drinking it daily, even sharing it with my dog (what's good for us humans has gotta be good for our best friends as well). Soon I began to notice a new-found energy and feeling of well-being. It didn't hit me all at once like those high-energy drinks do, but instead provided a slow and steady

increase in my vitality. Over time, I noted that I even stopped getting seasonal colds, and flu, and the bronchitis I had suffered frequent bouts of became a thing of the past.

I knew I was onto something and the following year, in 2010, I began processing and selling Chaga tea bags, (manually and painstakingly filling them by hand) and promoting them on my wood-products website. The sales started off slow as folks had no idea what it was, so consequently to generate interest and sales I ended up giving a lot of it away. Much of this went to friends and acquaintances, some of whom had been given severe and life-altering diagnosis, and it was quickly noticed that the addition of this tea to their diet was achieving remarkably beneficial results. The Chaga appeared to be making a huge difference to their wellbeing -- in some cases totally returning them to optimum good health. Then in 2012, as the word got out and sales increased, I added Chaga lip balm and skin crème to my products inventory, and created a website just for Chaga.

ENTER THE FDA

Having a presence online makes one an easy target for speculation and investigation, nevertheless I was astonished when one day I received a visit at my home (I was still conducting all my business activity from my home) from a moderately intimating uniformed FDA Agent. He introduced himself, and then stated that he was here to conduct an inspection. I immediately asked him if there was an issue with home-based businesses when it involved a 'food' product. His answer was 'absolutely not.' I quizzed him further. 'Then are you here because

186

someone made a complaint?' He nodded, 'Yes.' I immediately guessed that it had come from a former disgruntled sales rep that I had recently let go. He had been holding out for a larger share of the business and I had parted ways with him. He reacted by contacting the FDA and filed a complaint stating that our handling of Chaga was unsanitary. The agent verified that he was indeed the one who had filed the complaint. Fortunately, upon inspection, it was deemed that all was being handled properly and appropriately and we passed with 'flying colors'. Nevertheless, according to the Agent, our record keeping was weak and for that he issued a citation. I knew that every single step had to be accurately and precisely recorded while processing the product (if you scratch your head while packaging it - record it!) and I believed we had been doing an exemplary job of it. He also stated that the Chaga had to be labeled as a 'dietary supplement'. (I have since come to realize that that is not necessarily the case - if it does not cross state lines it does not have to be labeled a dietary supplement. If I sold Chaga only in the state of Maine the FDA would have no jurisdiction over it, but as I sell this stuff all over the world the FDA calls the shots) Well, the Agent instructed me to fill out a bevy of forms requiring the detailing of reams of information and send it all into their main office in Boston. This I did.

It was another two years before the next shoe dropped. FDA agents once again showed up at my home, and again in their slightly more intimidating uniforms, and once again conducted a full inspection. I just wasn't getting it. What were they looking for? What did they want from me? Apparently I was not doing certain things to their standards. I was mystified but when I asked them what more I needed to be doing, I was told that all the information I needed was available on their website and that I should look it up. Rightly so - all the verbiage was there - everything I needed to know to sell a 'dietary supplement'. Well . . . let me tell you . . . I'm familiar with law books, as I've spent years in law enforcement and was required to comply with the statues put forth by that genre, but when I started reading the multitude of FDA statues it put my head into a spin-cycle. My mind was boggled, the information was overwhelming complex and confusing. I was more mystified than before, and struggling to do my darnest to comply.

Then last year, in 2015, they again knocked on my door. Two agents with pressed uniforms showed up for a three-day visit. When these fellows arrive at your door your business comes to a complete halt. Everything stops while you provide them with all your records, give them 100% of your time, and the while sit calmly as they delve meticulously through every aspect of your business - while you ignore your ringing phone and put all your customer dealings on hold. You literally watch your business go 'down the tubes' for the duration of their visit. And this happened with each of the visits these guys made!

Then finally the curious mystery was revealed - the silence was broken, the veil was lifted, and these guys let slip their human side. It appears that there are very strict rules that apply to dietary supplements and these guys asked me why was I packaging my Chaga products as 'dietary supplements.' I answered that the first FDA Agent, back in 2012 told me that I must do so. These guys argued with me that this could not have been the case. I stepped back - said I would not argue with them - but swore that I was telling it like it was. Then came the shocker. One of the agents stepped forward and said quietly 'That's why we're here. That's the reason for all your visits. It's because you label your products as dietary supplements. It does not need to be. Oh, and by the way, neither can you site medical benefits nor post customer testimonials on your website.' They went still further explaining - in layman's terms (atypically for this agency) - exactly what was required of me. I finally got it. Yes, it is all about the paperwork. That's what it was from the beginning. But there's more. One of the agents lifted the veil still further, offering me the final solution. In a quiet aside he asked me if I knew any mycologists. Bingo! Of course I did. Even though I routinely sent my Chaga to a lab to be tested for any microbials, the FDA required that the Chaga be identified, verified and documented by a qualified mycologist. Why couldn't that have been made plain to me four years ago? So once I understood that was what they wanted from me, and had sought from the beginning, I immediately followed up and presented the Federal Drug Administration with a formal document from my mycologist stately absolutely that my Chaga was indeed Chaga and could be marketed as such. I took a deep breath - stopped running - and hopped off the 'hamster wheel'."

This entrepreneur wishes to remain anonymous.

IT COULD HAVE BEEN WORSE

Since 1973, Tahoma Clinic has provided effective treatments based Dr. Jonathan V. Wright, M.D., Medical Director and founder of the Tahoma Clinic. Dr. Wright is a pioneer in holistic medicine and bio-identical hormone replacement therapy. The Tahoma Clinic emphasizes the use of natural substances and natural energies for both the prevention and treatment of health problems not requiring surgical intervention.

"Our approach includes a personalized total-health evaluation to assess digestion, assimilation, metabolism, deficiencies, allergies and toxicities. Our 35 years of experience have taught us that a large number of symptoms and conditions unresponsive to conventional treatment – or only suppressed by patent medications – will yield to the application of Nature's remedies."

Dr. Wright's Story

"In 1992 a forceful contingent from the Kings County Sheriff's Office, acting as agents for the FDA, invaded my clinic WITH GUNS DRAWN! They were erroneously informed by the FDA that my clinic was selling DRUGS. This because our treatments were "outside their standard of care" (we were successfully treating patients with nature's natural remedies and vitamins. The FDA decrees that <u>anything</u> *given in the treatment of a patient is classified as a DRUG; therefore - according to them - my clinic utilizing holistic, natural substances and energies, was functioning as an illegal dealer, administrating and selling DRUGS! The King's County Sheriff's Department was totally operating under the misguided belief that they were conducting a full-fledge drug raid.*

At 9 am, with their guns drawn, they kicked in the doors of my clinic, and immediately pointed a gun directly at the head of my receptionist. Then they herded all my employees into a corner of the reception room, and proceeded to begin seizing equipment, medical records, payroll records, and even the clinic's banking records.

Eventually a grand jury was impaneled. We waited eighteen months and 'nothing' - no indictments. They impaneled a second grand jury and eighteen months later - still 'nothing' - again, no indictments. Then it was announced to the newspapers - not me, or my attorney - that they were closing the investigation. We stumbled upon this information in a back page newspaper article. We never got our patients records back, or our banking records. The latter we had to reconstruct as best we could. As for the former, with the patient's input, we eventually rebuilt each and every medical history record, but the damage to my practice was incalculable."

Here Dr. Wright refers to the "Fitzgerald Report," the result of an important investigation into the suspected conspiracy felt to be rampant in the medical business.
Read on -

"In the 1950's, Congressman Charles Tobey enlisted Benedict Fitzgerald, an investigator for the Interstate Commerce Commission, to investigate allegations of conspiracy and monopolistic practices on the part of orthodox medicine. This came about as the result of the son of Senator Tobey who developed cancer and was given less than two years to live by orthodox medicine. However, Tobey Jr., discovered options in the alternative field, received alternative treatment and fully recovered

from his cancerous condition! That is when he learned of alleged conspiratorial practices on the part of orthodox medicine. He passed the word to his father, Senator Charles Tobey, who initiated an investigation. The final report clearly indicated there was indeed a conspiracy to monopolize the medical and drug industry and to eliminate alternative options.

The "Fitzgerald Report" was submitted into the Congressional Record Appendix August 3, 1953.

Damning as this report is, congress never acted upon it. In addition, Congressman Tobey further identified the suspected conspiracy between the unholy trinity: The FDA, the patent medicine companies, and the AMA (American Medical Association) as being real and valid.

*****

"Pharmaceutical companies are the 'holders of patents' and have no place in the health care of the human body." ~ Dr. Nalini Chilkov, L.Ac., O.M.D., *Dr. Chilkov is a leading-edge authority on Integrative Cancer Care, Immune Enhancement, Optimal Nutrition and Wellness Medicine.*

*****

WELL, THE TIMING COULDN'T HAVE BEEN BETTER!

Just as these chapters were being written the press unveiled an outrage within the depths of the pharmaceutical industry - the EpiPen scandal!

Read on:

> "The EpiPen scandal has transformed Mylan Pharmaceuticals and its CEO Heather Bresch into the newest symbols of corporate greed."

"In the span of just a few weeks, they've gone from little-known players in the vast pharmaceutical industry to the targets of national ridicule over a relentless series of EpiPen price hikes."

Since 2009, Mylan has jacked up the price of the lifesaving allergy treatment an incredible 15 times. The list price on a two-pack of EpiPens is $609, up 400% from seven years ago.

The national outrage this month (Sept, 2016), sparked by a social media campaign by parents, has forced Mylan to respond by taking the unusual step of launching a generic version of EpiPen at a 50% discount to its current price, as well as other moves to make the treatment more affordable.

Despite those efforts, Congress is now investigating Mylan. The powerful House Oversight Committee sent a letter to CEO Bresch on Monday requesting a briefing and a trove of documents from the company about EpiPen.

Mylan has sought to pin the blame for the sticker shock on the shadowy health care supply chain. Bresch called the system "broken" and said it was in a "crisis," similar to the financial crisis of 2008 that blew up the economy."

Here's another outrage:

The drug Daraprim, essential for AIDS and transplant patients, cost just $13.50/per pill in 2009. Now in 2016 the price is a staggering $750.00/per pill. Further irony, this same pill can be bought outside the U.S. for $1.00. Originally marketed by Impax Laboratories, Inc., in August of 2015 they recently announced the sale of Daraprim to Turing Pharmaceuticals AG for $55 million.

And on a more personal note:

This writer must use a prescribed Premarin product for a rather delicate (and not to be disclosed) female issue. The product comes in a tube which contains 0.625mg/g of the stuff. Each time the prescription is filled (approximately every 4 months) I've noted a $10.00 price increase. In Nov. 2014 the cost (without insurance factored in) was $149.26 per tube. In May of this year (2016) the cost had risen to a whopping $208.38. Premarin is manufactured from the urine of a pregnant mare and the patent is held exclusively by Wyeth Pharmaceuticals, Inc. (A subsidiary of Pfizer, Inc.)

*****

So . . . what is the consumer and patient to do?

"No disease can exist inside of a clean body."
~ Dr. Edward F. Group III, D.C., N.D.
CEO of Global Healing Center,
Speaker, Author, & Educator.

Chapter *Twenty two*

"No disease can exist inside of a clean body."

SO HOW DOES ONE ATTAIN A CLEAN BODY?

Our current food supply is morally bankrupt. We've got a food system that is full of flavorings, and additives, and chemicals, and colors, and genetically modified organisms, and pesticides, and hormones, and antibiotics. All of these things together are creating a toxic soup and this toxic soup is slowly killing us. It's leading to staggering two-thirds of our population suffering from obesity, with a third of our kids expected to get diabetes within their lifetimes, plus massive epidemics of cancer.

We didn't know 50 or 60 years ago the role that the immune system played like we do today because we didn't have the technology to measure and identify it. In order for having a maximum chance of fighting and overcoming illnesses, diseases and cancer, we need an intact immune system. That, too, makes the current approach of chemotherapy so unethical. It destroys the immune system, and the first organ that is affected, actually the target organ, is the bone marrow. WHAT TO DO?

FIRST ~ Plant a garden:

The garden should actually be better considered as a pharmacy. Your food is your cure and your prime medicine: We're not designed to be ingesting or be exposed to molecules that aren't from nature. It is an absolute fact that the food you put in your body has an enormous impact on your genetic expression. This has been proven beyond a doubt through the sciences of Nutrigenomics and Igenetics. *(These are the sciences that study the interaction of nutrition on genes, with regard to the prevention and treatment of diseases. Their findings hold great promise in fighting obesity, cancers and all other life-altering diseases, and have transformed the way we think about genomes.).*

I can hear you all shutter and stammer . . . "I live in an apartment!" . . . "I have no yard!" . . . "I know nothing about gardening!"

Well, even a small patch of ground - possibly a raised garden - or collection of large planters sopping up the sun on terraces and porches would imply a start toward "eating green". Other very viable sources are your local farm stand, farmer's markets, health food stores and even communal and co-op gardens - but do your research and buy from only those who grow their crops organically - no pesticides no herbicides, no chemical fertilizers. These things were not meant to put in our bodies. And why is this important?

Today we are overwhelmed with hype of all kinds and perhaps the one most needed to be questioned is the consumption of foods labeled (or not labeled) GMO's (Genetically Modified Organisms). Many health groups say there are unanswered questions regarding the potential long-term impact on human health from food derived from GMOs. Concerns include contamination of the non-genetically modified food supply, effects of GMOs on the environment and nature, the rigor of the regulatory process, and consolidation of control of the food supply in companies that make and sell GMOs, or concerns over the use of herbicides with glyphosate (a chemical used in weed killer) The issue of safety has swirled around GMOs since genetic researchers first introduced them in the 1970s. While proponents have heralded the almost-limitless potential of GMOs to fight disease, improve crop yields and safeguard the environment, critics have decried the development of genetically tweaked "Frankenfoods" that could spread from agricultural fields into the rest of the environment, with potentially catastrophic ecological results. Among the critics' most serious charges are GMOs' potential to stimulate the rise of antibiotic-resistant "superbugs" and pesticide-resistant "superweeds" that require the use of increasingly powerful drugs and hazardous chemicals. There's also evidence that GMOs are largely used to increase profits for agribusiness interests at the expense of smaller farmers who do not use GMO crops. Don't mess with nature.

(Put a handful of Epsom salts in a gallon of water and introduce it into the soil supporting your plants and trees. You'll be surprised at the enhanced flavors it will generate.)

THEN ~ Eat a Rainbow:
(The brighter and more vibrant the color - the sweeter and more advantageous the results)
RED: Apples, beetroot, red cabbage, cherries, cranberries, red potatoes, red bell peppers, radishes, strawberries, tomatoes and watermelon.
These help keep your heart and bladder healthy and your memory strong.

ORANGE and YELLOW: Apricots, pumpkin, carrots, mangoes, nectarines, oranges, papayas, peaches, yellow pears, pineapples, sweet corn, sweet potatoes, tangerines, yellow bell peppers.

These foods help keep your heart and eyes healthy and boost your immune system.

GREEN: Asparagus, avocados, green beans, broccoli, brussel sprouts, green cabbage, spinach, zucchini, celery, kiwifruit, cucumbers, lettuce, green pears.

These help keep your eyes healthy and your bones and teeth strong.

PURPLE: Blackberries, black currents, blueberries, plums and prunes, eggplant, purple grapes and purple potatoes.

These aid in overall good health and help prevent colds and flu while keeping your bladder and memory strong.

BROWN and WHITE: Bananas, brown pears, cauliflower, garlic, onions, mushrooms, white potatoes, turnips, white nectarines, shallots, parsnips, white nectarines, ginger and dates.

These help keep your heart healthy and encourage good cholesterol levels.

AND DON'T FORGET THE SEEDS AND NUTS!

Seeds and nuts are tremendously valuable because they carry little packets of concentrates, nutrients, about 20 to 30 fold more than the rest of the fruit, so it's a fabulous packet of concentrated nutrition. They've got all sorts of genetic spare parts that can spring into action to grow into a plant, or tree, to become a vehicle capable of repairing our DNA and our RNA[1] It also has tremendous stem cell precursors, especially in the husk of seeds and nuts.

Consider the benefits of substituting your current flour and bread products with ancient grains. Here's a few to consider: millet, barley, bulgur, buckwheat, oats, chia, and quinoa.

AND THEN THERE'S JUICING

Put that blender to work that's sitting idly on the counter. Throw in some kale, wheatgrass[2] a few baby carrots, cucumbers, celery, a tomato, a bit of broccoli, a healthy dollop of yogurt, a little ginger, and a generous splash of Chaga tea and/or juice and whip it all up! Your body can begin to absorb it right away, because it's going to go right into your system. It is at work in your system in about 20 or 30 minutes, bringing that life directly into your body, and binding up all those toxins and getting them ready to be carried right out of the body.

ELIMINATE ALL SUGARS

Yes, I know you have a 'sweet tooth', an unquenchable need for all things sweet. So do I. It may be the hardest thing of all to eliminate from your daily diet but, once you begin to consume those non-chemically raised fruits, and vegetables, right off the vine, out of the earth, dead ripe and bursting with the goodness of their natural sugars you should, and will, be satisfied. Give them a chance. And those sugar substitutes like Splenda and Aspartame and Sucratose? Avoid them like the plague! On the other hand, Stevia has been deemed a safe substitute for sugar. It is derived from the leaves of the stevia plant and is considered a herb or dietary supplement.

THROW AWAY YOUR DEODORANT:

I'm not condoning a smelly existence but if your current deodorant contains aluminum get rid of it! Several years ago, during an annual mammogram the technician voiced her opinion that the reason for the modern-day proliferation of breast cancer might be the aluminum that is in most deodorant products, and the proximity of the armpit to the breast. I threw mine away and have exclusively used TOM'S of MAINE ever since - no aluminum - and no smell!

NEXT ~ Learn all there is to know about essential oils, herbs and vitamins:

Become familiar with specific herbs, supplements, vitamins and essential oils as they have proven themselves throughout history to effect and enhance mankind's health and wellbeing. Become skilled at knowing how to use them to achieve the best results for you.

Essential oils are a volatile organic compound. There are no nutrition values in them, nor are there any vitamins or minerals. They are chemicals that essentially nature gave to plants to protect them from outside threats, whether it is bacteria, viruses, fungus or infectors such as flies, bees - or whatever else that might attack the plant.

There are so many oils, herbs and vitamins to consider, but those listed here give you a head start on becoming familiar with some of the more well-known and revered.

Frankincense oil: Probably the most powerful essential oil if not the most powerful supplement, period, when it comes to natural cancer treatment and very effective against Alzheimer's.

Myrrh: This powerhouse works on the hypothalamus in the liver. It reduces liver inflammation and also balances hormones.

Lemon oil: Used for virtually everything: detoxification, internally, externally – whether you use it to clean the counter, or to clean your skin. It also proves effective for everything from nausea to halitosis to diabetes.

Peppermint oil: For everything, including sparking the creative juices. Soak a cotton ball in peppermint and set it next to the space where you sit while creating the next "'Great American Novel" or the County Fair's next prize-winning piece of art and feel your creativity soar.

Eucalyptus oil: This oil has long been known to benefit the respiratory system

Tea Tree Essential Oil: The health benefits attributed to this oil are its properties as an antibacterial, antimicrobial, antiseptic, antiviral, balsamic, expectorant, fungicide, insecticide and stimulant.

Turmeric: Middle Easterners use turmeric in cancer treatments.

Lavender and Sandalwood: these two have proven incredible at fighting cancer

Resveratrol : A type of natural phenol, and phytoalexin produced naturally by several plants in response to injury or when the plant is under attack by pathogens such as bacteria or fungi. Sources of resveratrol in food include the skin of grapes, blueberries, raspberries, and mulberries. Used as a dietary supplement, it has been noted that high doses of resveratrol produce statistically significant reductions in systolic blood pressure, and stimulates bone formation.

Chaga: The Chaga in all its forms, the tincture, the balm, the lotion, the tea are beneficial to nearly every part, every organ, and all the workings of your entire body.

VITAMINS

Your body needs vitamins to operate at its optimal level. Two distinct kinds of vitamins exist: fat-soluble and water-soluble. Fat-soluble vitamins consist of vitamins A, E, D and K, while water-soluble vitamins include the B vitamins and vitamin C. All these vitamins perform particular jobs in your body and benefit your health in a multitude of ways

Vitamin A helps maintain good eyesight and supports normal growth of cells. By maintaining adequate intakes of vitamin A, you can keep your teeth, bones, skin and mucus membranes and immune system in good health.

Vitamin B complex is comprised of eight vitamins, which include B-1, B-2, B-3, B-5, B-6, B-7, B-12 and folate, or B-9. These vitamins help your body produce the energy it needs to function better and assists in the formation of red blood cells.

Vitamin C is an antioxidant. Vitamin C protects your body against the effects of free radicals, unstable molecules that damage your DNA and may enhance the aging process and the development of health issues such as arthritis, cancer and heart disease. Vitamin C is responsible for the growth and repair of body tissues and for repairing and maintaining bones and teeth and for healing wounds. Chaga is the most powerful source of antioxidants.

Vitamin D: Evidence suggests that this vitamin may reduce your risk of certain cancers, particularly of the pancreas, breast, prostate, colon and skin, and it provides protection from osteomalacia, the softening of bones in adults. You can get a fairly respectable amount of vitamin D from exposure to sunlight.

Vitamin E: The antioxidant properties of this vitamin protect your body from free radical damage and helps boost your immune system, enabling it to battle bacterial and viral infections. It helps your body use vitamin K, the blood-clotting vitamin and also contributes to the formation of red blood cells.

Vitamin K: Your body stores vitamin K in the liver and fat tissue. It plays an important role in helping blood clot properly and it also helps your body use calcium to build bone, encouraging the development of healthy bones and decreasing the risk of bone fractures

IMPORTANT ~ Balance Your Energy:

As an energetic being, reflect on all you can do to keep your electricity and energy flowing properly. A few additions to your regime that will guide and support you along in your quest for a sound and happy body are chiropractic care, acupuncture, exercise, the proper amount of sleep, and making sure that your hormones are in balance. And get off that couch! Strive to walk 7000, to 10,000 steps a day and while out there soak up some of that good vitamin D, courtesy of the sun. Want a fun and creative way to relieve stress? One sure-fired cure is the new coloring books for grownups. This phenomenon cropped up earlier this year, and has swept the country catching the imagination of adults the world over. They're available just about everywhere. Try one. You'll be glad you did.

THEN ~ Detox:

We are living in a toxic world where trees are dying, the soil is sick, the water, and even the very air we breathe is contaminated. So what can we do about it? How do we make, and keep, our bodies clean? We start by reducing our toxic exposure. Read the labels on the products you are using. Weed killers, laundry detergents, supermarket foods, household cleaners, cosmetics, shampoos, everything else should be subject to scrutiny. Look for alternatives to these products i.e: vinegar can be a prime ingredient in cleaning your home. (Look it up - lots of info on the internet about this) There are specific things that you can do to help support the detoxification pathways in your body and to prevent those toxins from entering into your body in the first place.

Again: ***Read all labels of every item in your home.***

The process of detoxification is multistep and takes a commitment on the part of the follower as it is spread over a significant period of time. The steps can be a bit convoluted, so for the purposes of this book I shall condense and simplify them. There are reams of information on this course of action written by credible and knowledgeable followers of this procedure which the reader is encouraged to research further. Here are the basics:

1. Clean the colon. One suggested approach is colon hydrotherapy utilizing herbal supplements and herbs psyllium, bentonite, slippery elm bark, humic acid and - yes - even coffee enemas.

2. The next step would be to detox the urinary tract, the kidneys, and bladder. Start with drinking lots of water, add parsley and asparagus in larger-then-usual amounts to your diet, and top it off with marshmallow root.

3. Then should be the liver. A few of the suggested ways are: turmeric, milk thistle, virtually all of your root vegetables (beets, ginger, burdock) and again, a coffee enema is suggested as well as drinking olive oil with Epsom salts (a very old approach).

4. The lymph nodes would be the last thing to focus on. Among the possible cleansers include cat's claw, burdock root, and Essiac formula.

5. Then comes a parasite cleanse. A proper parasite cleanse takes six weeks because that's the cycle of most parasites from the time that they lay eggs until the time they are an adult. Suggestions for this include black walnut hull, American wormseed, clove, kamala, and that combination with a couple of other ones with Bromelain, Epazote, Diatomaceous earth and perhaps a bit of clove. A simpler solution is the daily use of Chaga.

6. The sixth one is foods. Read, analyze, and become absolutely certain of the food products you are putting into your body. The irradiation, the homogenization, the pasteurization, the genetic modification of foods, all change the basic molecular structure of those foods that we're taking into our body just to sustain ourselves. These overly processed foods are severely detrimental to the body.

7. Spiritual Toxicity: Learn to nurture and love yourself. Forgive yourself and others for past indiscretions. Learn to manage your stress and let go of the past and never bottle up those negative emotions inside of you. They will fester and cause you to experience poor health. When old emotional wounds and spiritual pains surface, and it seems more than you can handle, it's a good idea to seek professional help to aid in the detoxification process. EFT[3], and emotional trauma therapy may also help you to let go of your emotional pain. The detoxification of the emotional and spiritual level in conjunction with the physical level are tightly linked together and should be treated as such. Stress, mental anguish, negative thoughts and emotions are all detrimental to health, setting the stage for all kinds of diseases and mal-functions to arrive upon the scene. Stress diminishes the immune system because it increases cortical, which suppresses the immune system, thereby depleting melatonin, vitamin C, and niacin. A negative thought can kill you faster than a bad germ. It's been proven that the body can heal itself with just positive visualization. There are records of cancer patients having used simple visualization, experiencing a total cure. Or . . . you can.

GET A PET:

Studies have shown that petting your dog or cat reduces your blood pressure by 10 to 20 millimeters. There is nothing better for you, your mental health and overall wellbeing than, at the end of a stressful day, to be greeted by a dog imparting wet kisses, tail wags and manifesting all the joy unconditional love can muster.

OH - and by the way - **Find a holistic[4] dentist** and go on a regular basis:

Your teeth have a much larger impact on your health than you might ever have imagined. They are connected to your organs through your meridian system. What may be lurking in your teeth, gums and mouth will affect your health. If your mouth is harboring toxic amalgams, it's a given that it's causing toxicity in the body. What it boils down to is that every one of the 32 spots in the jaw are directly connected to organs in our body, whether there is a tooth there or not. This connection is quite intimate and if you're using toothpaste containing fluoride (and most do) throw it in the trash. According to a 2011 article in *Time Magazine* they listed as one of the top ten most toxic household chemicals - *Fluoride* - It disrupts the metabolism of other key elements that are needed for healthy bone growth. It activates the osteosarcoma genes, increasing the possibility of leukemia, and perhaps other bone-based cancers. Those genes become activated by elevated fluoride levels in our bodies. A good alternative? TOM'S of MAINE provides the consumer with a fluoride-free tooth paste and mouthwash.

Of special note: the FLUORIDE in your drinking water is slowly destroying the pineal gland through calcification. This gland is vital for a healthy immune system. Melanin-enriched Chaga is key in restoring this gland to optimum function.

"Modern conventional medicine battles disease directly by means of drugs, surgery, radiation and other therapies, but true health can only be attained by maintaining a healthy, properly functioning immune system."

Phyllis A. Balch, CNC & James F. Balch, M.D.

[1] Ribonucleic acid is a polymeric molecule essential in various biological roles in coding, decoding, regulation, and expression of genes.

[2] Wheat grass contains chlorophyll, amino acids, minerals, vitamins, and enzymes. Claims about the health benefits of wheatgrass range from providing supplemental nutrition to having unique curative properties.

[3] EFT is the practice of using positive affirmations while tapped into certain acupuncture points, thereby releasing the painful and replacing them with new and refreshing substitutes.

[4] A Holistic dentist provides dental treatment with a natural approach; for example, repairing teeth with non-toxic materials. This method of dentistry is known as environmental or biological dentistry.

Chapter *Twenty three*

BACK TO THE WOODS

I left Florida in late June - before the oppressive heat could overwhelm me. It was my season for Chaga hunting and I couldn't wait to enter into the dark, cool woods of Northern Maine, Vermont and New Hampshire. I would be there for nearly three months, hopefully long enough to have bypassed all those long, hot, steamy dog days of summer in Central Florida. Terry would stay behind and tend the cats, set up and market Chaga at all our various venues, and do all those things necessary to keep our solar dome functioning properly. She would join me in early October and together we would make the trip back down to the southlands. All happened as planned and we arrived back home just after hurricane Matthew made a swipe at Florida's east coast. Fortunately, he was kind to us and left no structural damage in his wake - only messy blow downs to pick up after.

As usual I had packed enough gear to sustain myself in the woods for a three months stay. My Hennessy Hammock, mountain bike and kayak hunkered familiarly against and atop my 1985 Mercedes and rounded out my arsenal. My itinerary, going north, included stopovers along the way in favorite nooks on the Appalachian Trail. Those first nights away from Florida's oppressive heat, sleeping in the great outdoors were beyond refreshing, they were down-right frigid! I shivered, shook and piled on a few extra layers of flannel.

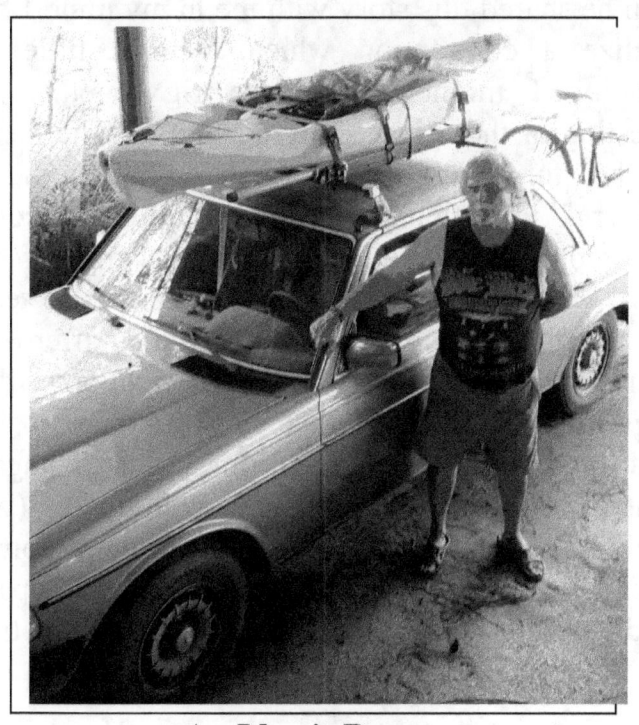

An Idea is Born

Sometime after we had ended our Rainbow Spring ventures my old buddy "Fishin' Fred" became enamored with a lady hiker from Vermont. During the courtship, and his frequent visits to The Green Mountain State to court her, he would stay at a rustic camp ground near the southern terminus of the Green Mountains, just off the Appalachian Trail. Many evenings, he would sit by the campfire and stare up into the nighttime skies. As his eyes wandered he suddenly realized that he was starring at an *enormous* Chaga, 40 feet up the side of a nearby birch tree. Fishin' Fred knew just what he was looking at and the value it represented, both monetarily and health-wise, but at 40 feet from the ground it was nearly impossible to harvest. Any attempt would be a threat to life and limb. When he shared this story with me in my mind I began to visualize a contraption which, with a little Yankee ingenuity, I might be able to rig together for the harvesting of these inaccessible beauties. The idea began to take form and shape and an awesome "Rube Goldberg"[1] invention was born. This apparatus consists of many repurposed and restructured odd mix of bits and pieces. Once rigged together I was anxious to test it out and hopefully this year's hunt would offer me that opportunity. I had only to find the right tree, the right Chaga and yes, the one that was taunting me from its heretofore unreachable perch. Prior to this a Chaga hunter might resort to climbing the tree with spikes (which is definitely not good for the tree) or attempt some other madcap scenario which could result in his corpse being found years hence dangling awkwardly from the tree.

~ ~ ~ ~ ~ ~

My first stop on my northward trek was in the Nantahala Mountains of western North Carolina. This was not so much to seek out Chaga as to take a few days to recuperate from the unrelenting heat I'd just escaped. From there I headed toward the Green Mountains in Vermont and met up with Mark, an old Chaga-hunting friend. Together we ventured deep into the mountains specifically seeking those elusive Chagas that had taunted us in the past from their lofty heights. Together we tested out my new invention and found it to work very effectively.

From the "Greens" I progressed into the "Whites" of New Hampshire and eventually ended up in Western Maine. While passing through Gorham, New Hampshire, the headquarters for the White Mountain National Forest, I had the opportunity to talk with one of their representatives. I needed to know if what I was doing, harvesting Chaga, was allowed in New Hampshire's National Forests. I was assured that there were no restrictions against this or for that matter, any type of foraging. This came as a bit of a surprise but also as a relief knowing that I could continue my quest among these majestic forested mountains.

As it turned out, I was experiencing one of the best harvests of my Chaga hunting career. With approximately 50 to 60 pounds of the mushrooms, I headed eastward into the cool and magnificent forests of northern Maine.

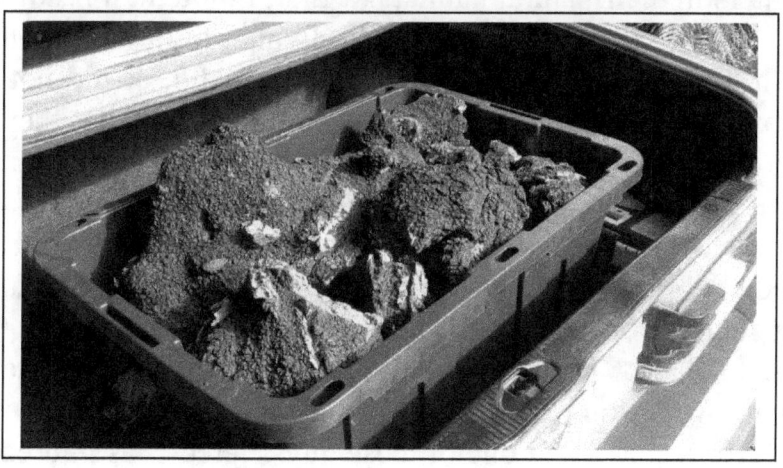

Once there I settled in at a primitive campsite at the edge of a pristine river hung out my survival hammock and prepared to take a 'breather.' I rested, napped, read, and just enjoyed the heck out of this quiet respite beside this glorious body of water.

A few days into this, as I was feeling refreshed, restored, and nearly ready to begin the next leg of my journey, I heard an approaching vehicle. Very shortly thereafter, a pickup truck pulled in next to my campsite and a couple of young fellas proceeded to pitch a tent and set up camp. (Please note: I refer to anybody less old than I as 'young'. Actually they were probably in their late 30's, early 40's.) I couldn't help but overhear their banter and I kept hearing the word "Chaga". Of course my antenna activated and I went into high alert.

I rolled out of my hammock and made my way over to them with hand outstretched and introduced myself. They in turn identified themselves as Jared and Billy and told me they were Chaga hunters. I smiled to myself thinking it curious to meet up with other Chaga hunters in their natural habitat. At first, I thought it best to just listen, play dumb, and not to divulge my association with Chaga. I wanted to learn what they did, or did not, know about this pursuit. I soon came to realize that they were still pretty green. So as these fellas went on about Chaga I would occasionally interject a bit of my own knowledge. I had them puzzled - no doubt about it - and it made me chuckle just a bit. Finally, looking at me in puzzlement one of them said "You seem to know a lot about Chaga." Then I shook their hands again, and said to them, "Well you just met an Old Chaga Hunter."

I realized that one of these guys, Jared, was injured and seemingly rather badly. His t-shirt was bloodied and wrapped tightly about his shoulder. When he saw me looking at it he admitted that he had hurt himself and asked if I had any alcohol to clean it out. Naturally I wanted to know what happened and cringed as they related the story. This guy was lucky to be alive!

Jared began: They had spotted a handsome Chaga specimen about 15 feet up the side of a birch tree. As

Billy was the smaller of the two, it fell to him to climb upon Jared's shoulders - with ax in hand - in an attempt to reach it. From this precarious perch, and stretched to his limit, he swung the ax into the Chaga. But alas - the ax became deeply wedged into the mushroom. In an attempt to pull it free, it slipped from his grip and landed, cutting blade down, directly onto Jared's shoulder and tearing right through to the bone. *Good Lord! It could have been his head!*

Fortunately, when I go into the woods I carry with me a pretty well-stocked first aide kit. With those resources we were able to clean out the wound, pull it back together and secure it with butterfly closures - and all without any anesthesia. (Those Maine boys were tough!)

Well, having much in common, it was natural to share the evening campfire and reminisce about our experiences. Over a supper of fresh-caught salmon I easily slid into the role of teacher and Chaga guru. There was so much they didn't know and like sponges, they eagerly sopped up everything I had to say.

At first I was a bit reluctant to share information about my "invention" - the one that could bring down a Chaga from 40 feet up. It's a 'trade secret' I told them and I don't plan to divulge its design even in the book I'm writing. However, as the evening wore on I began to relate details about its design and virtues. They were eager to have a look and try it out.

Well, I liked these guys. They both were family men with young kids back home - and I felt sorry for their bad luck, and the accident that could have taken a life. So . . . I agreed to do a demonstration - if they found the perfect Chaga on the ideal tree at the optimum height.

So the next morning they were up bright and early and impatient to get on with the demonstration. The venture started out a bit precariously as we had to ford a section of the river to reach an island that seemed to be teeming with birch trees. The rocks were darn slippery and the current precarious. As I made my way across, I was definitely having second thoughts about this whole undertaking. However, we reached the island safely and began the search for the tree that would deliver to us the proper Chaga for our test. Well, we didn't find it so again wadded back over those slippery rocks, fortunately with no mishaps. I was ready to end the venture.

However, Billy was not so easily thwarted and he offered up a bribe that was hard to refuse. From the bed of their pickup he unwrapped the results of their Chaga hunt. I was impressed. Novices they might be but they had gathered an impressive harvest. Billy pointed to two of the biggest and best specimens and said; "If you show us how to harvest Chaga 40 feet up a tree without leaving the ground we'll give you these two pieces."
I was hooked, I swore them to secrecy, and with that I gathered up the implements of my invention, and proceeded to demonstrate just how it would work in a real situation. They were impressed.

We parted company the following day - both the richer for having spent time together.

~ ~ ~ ~ ~ ~

Since then, my invention has proved itself again and again. Mark has frequently joined me on my treks up to the North Country. Over the years we've done a lot of camping, hiking, and kayaking together. When I became involved in hunting Chaga (which admittedly is not just my livelihood but also an excuse, a purpose, to be in the deep woods that I love) I would frequently invite Mark to link up with me. He would pack up his truck, point it westerly and drive from Maine into the White Mountains of New Hampshire or the Green's of Vermont and we would set up a camp together. Now, with my 'invention' in tow, in tandem we would canvas the woods seeking those elusive Chagas, which beckoned us tantalizingly from 40 feet above our heads. My apparatus served us well as it performed at its finest when used by a two-man team.

~ ~ ~ ~ ~ ~

This was the first year of my Chaga hunting quests that I did not find these gems relatively visible and easily accessible along the more traveled hiking paths and trails. There was ample evidence that there had once been Chaga on these trees - but no longer. Any Chaga to be had in these easily reached locales had been harvested out. It is the fear - and prophecy - of many that the Chaga is in danger of going the way of the wild ginseng, and we will loose this natural resource within our lifetime. My belief is far more optimistic than that. I know there are hundreds of thousands of acres far deep in these forests that have not been tapped. Most folks, and that includes most fledging Chaga hunters, are not proficient in reading a compass, following a USGS Survey map, or in utilizing their GPS well enough to bushwhack their way about in those deep unfamiliar, and oft time hostile, forests of our North County. Those birches with their remarkable medicinal gifts are simply not easily reached by the untrained and unschooled casual hunter. To the betterment of mankind they will therefore remain relatively safe as an untapped resource; available to mankind for generations yet to come.

[1] *Reuben Garrett Lucius "Rube" Goldberg (July 4, 1883 – December 7, 1970) was an American cartoonist, sculptor, author, engineer, and inventor. Goldberg was best known for a series of popular cartoons depicting complicated gadgets that perform simple tasks in indirect, convoluted ways*

Chapter Twenty four

Black Mangroves
A Serendipitous Meeting
and
A NEW CHAGA PRODUCT IS BORN

There are about 80 different species of mangrove trees. All of these trees grow in areas with low-oxygen soil, where slow-moving waters allow fine sediments to accumulate. Mangrove forests only grow at tropical and subtropical latitudes near the equator because they cannot withstand freezing temperatures.

Many mangrove forests can be recognized by their dense tangle of prop roots that make the trees appear to be standing on stilts above the water. This tangle of roots allows the trees to handle the daily rise and fall of tides, which means that most mangroves get flooded at least twice per day. The roots also slow the movement of tidal waters, causing sediments to settle out of the water and build up the muddy bottom.

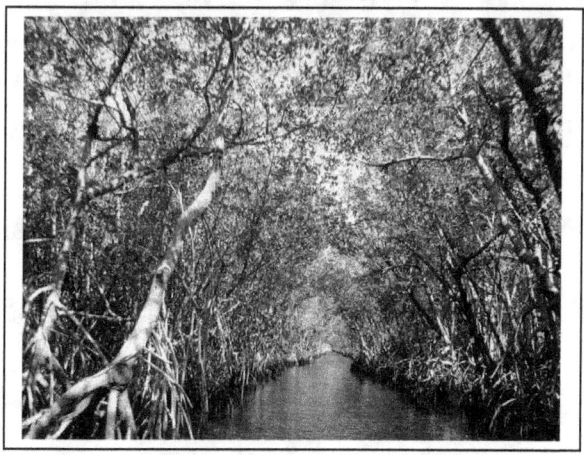

Mangrove forests stabilize the coastline, reducing erosion from storm surges, currents, waves, and tides. The intricate root system of mangroves also makes these forests attractive to fishes and other organisms seeking food and shelter from predators.

Mangroves line more than 1,800 miles of shoreline within Florida Keys National Marine Sanctuary. In the Florida Keys, the red mangrove, black mangrove, and white mangrove tend to dominate wetland areas.

The mangroves that I'm going to tell you about here grow pretty close to home, along Florida's famed intercostal waterways, in and around Mosquito Bay.

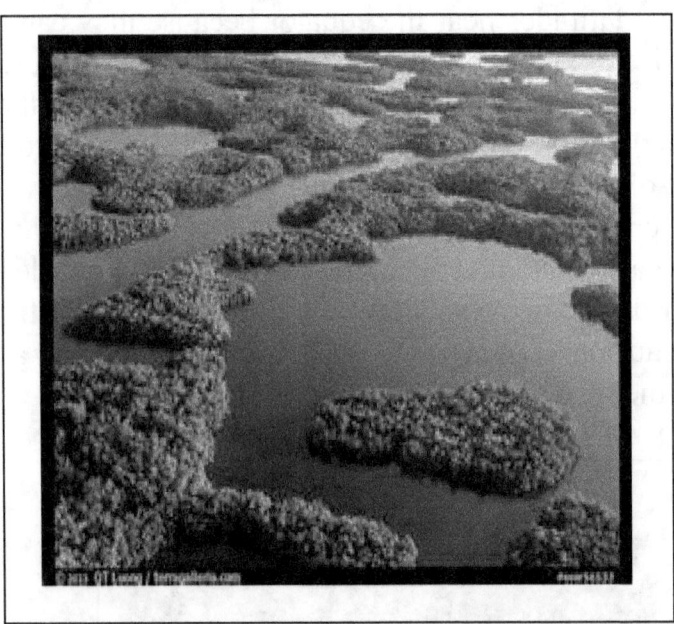

Earlier this spring, while tending my Chaga booth in New Smyrna, a young man named Christopher approached me showing great interest in my products. He asked all the right questions and then before we parted he told me he was involved in the process of gathering and marketing local honey derived from mangrove trees. I wished him well, and then thought no more about it.

Then this past fall, just after returning from my annual Chaga hunt, my wife and I were back on our usual circuit and were setting up at New Smyrna. I was approached again by Christopher who had shared his honey story months earlier, and he presented me with a sample of the stuff. After tasting it, I thought that it was perhaps the best honey I'd ever put in my mouth.

Well, it seems that Christopher is an associate of Sonny Yambor, owner of Sun Splash of New Smyrna Beach. This company had obtained the first ever permit from the Florida Department of the Environmental Protection for the placement of 2000 bee hives within the intercostal waterway region. The purpose of this joint agreement would allow for the harvesting of honey derived exclusively from the region's black mangroves.

Every summer since 2012, he's placed his hives on islands in the Indian River, around Mosquito Lagoon where mangroves are just about the only plants to blossom in the sweltering heat. The premise of the placement is that a bee only flies about a mile from the hive. So you situate the hives right in the middle of the river - with full access to the black mangrove giving the bee exclusive entrée to the lovely black mangrove flower. It seems that because the center depth of this flower is far more shallow then those of other mangrove flower varieties (the red and white) the bees have easier access to its nectar. It's a win-win

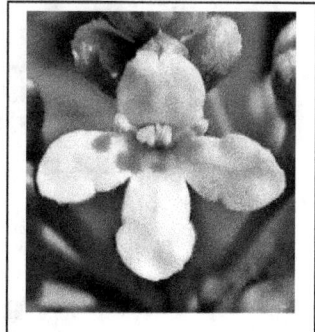

for all and it yields the best-tasting honey in the world with a velvety, thin texture and floral scent.

"The harvesting task isn't easy" says Yambor. "The boxy hives — about 1,600 of them this year — are not light, even before the bees fill them with 50 pounds of honey or more. Most of the colony sites are accessible only by water, which means loading about half of the hives onto and off a boat rather than a truck."

Yambor and his crew of six deliver them to the various sites as soon as the mangroves start blooming, which is generally the last week of May. The bees, about 50,000 per colony, spend their summer days flitting from one mangrove blossom to another, spreading pollen along their way aiding greatly in the propagation of the native vegetation.

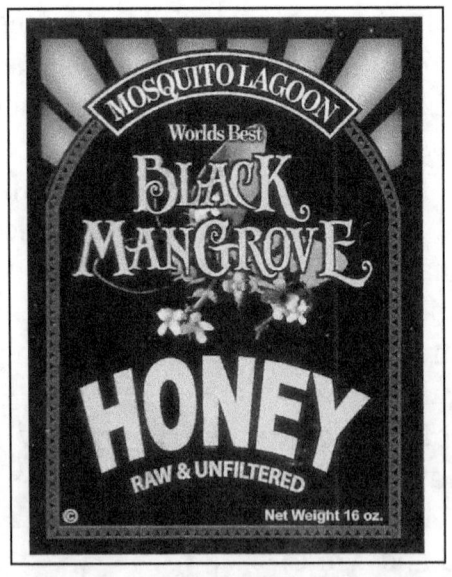

Yambor's
Sun Splash of New Smyrna
Beach.

Florida suffered a hard freeze during the winter of 1985-86 and nearly killed off these mangrove trees. It was the same winter that we lost the Challenger due to a frozen 0-ring, a devastating time for Florida in so many ways. It has taken all this time for them to make a full comeback. But they're back and thriving once again.

Of significant importance is the relationship of the black mangrove honey to human beings. These trees on which these blossoms grow derive their nutrients from the brackish backwater at the oceans edge. Harken back to Rachael Carson's *"The Sea Around Us"* when she relates *". . .each of us carries in our veins a salty stream in which the elements are combined in almost the same proportions as in sea water."* The briny environment sustaining and nurturing these trees is rich in the same salty proportion as that which flows through the veins of mankind. Honey derived from this source is specifically rich in all the trace minerals that sustain human life.

Now . . . historically Chaga has been infused into various types of honey in the past but never with black mangrove honey! What a boon to humankind that marriage would be! A delightful taste, easy to consume and full of all the life sustaining properties that both the Chaga and the black mangrove bring to the table.

So - a deal was struck and a partnership of sorts was created between Sonny Yambor, his Sun Splash of New Smyrna Beach Co. and me. He supplying the honey and I infusing it with Chaga. I believe this may be the first Chaga infused black mangrove honey the world has ever seen and Chaga Golden has it! An enormously important new superfood!

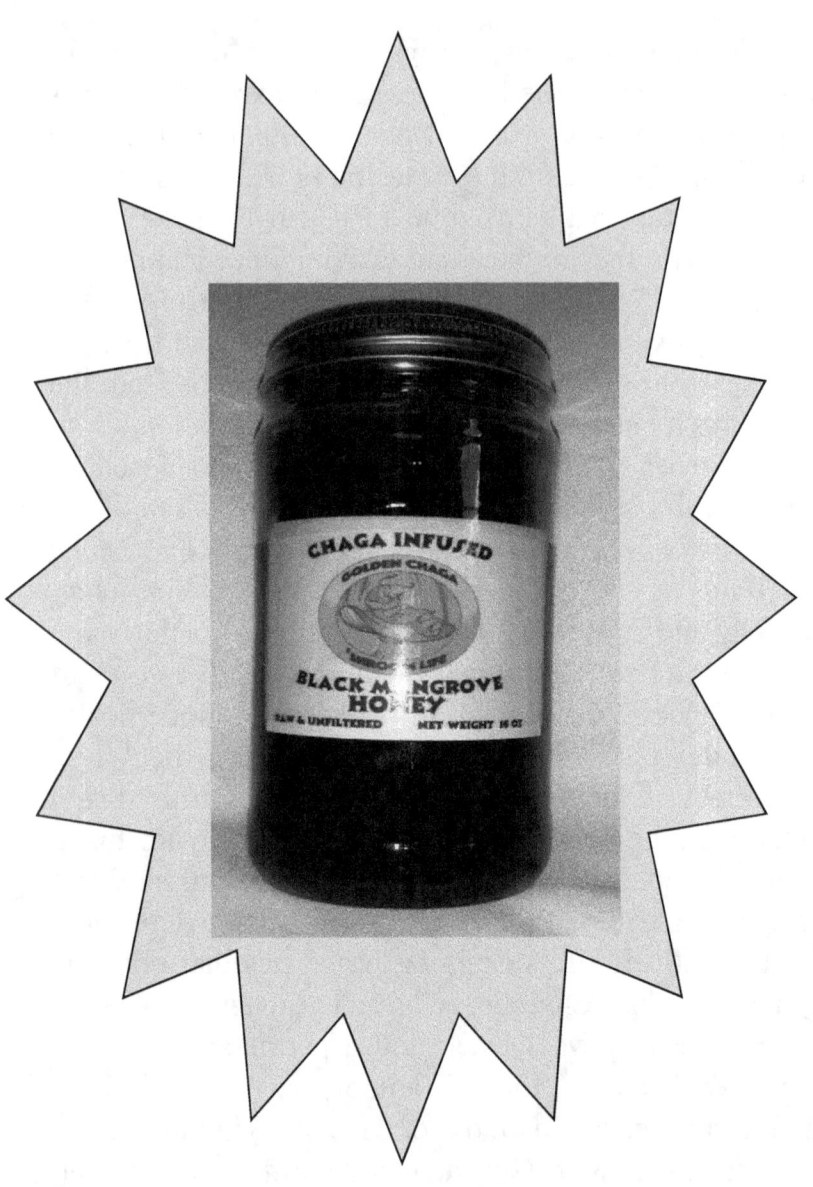

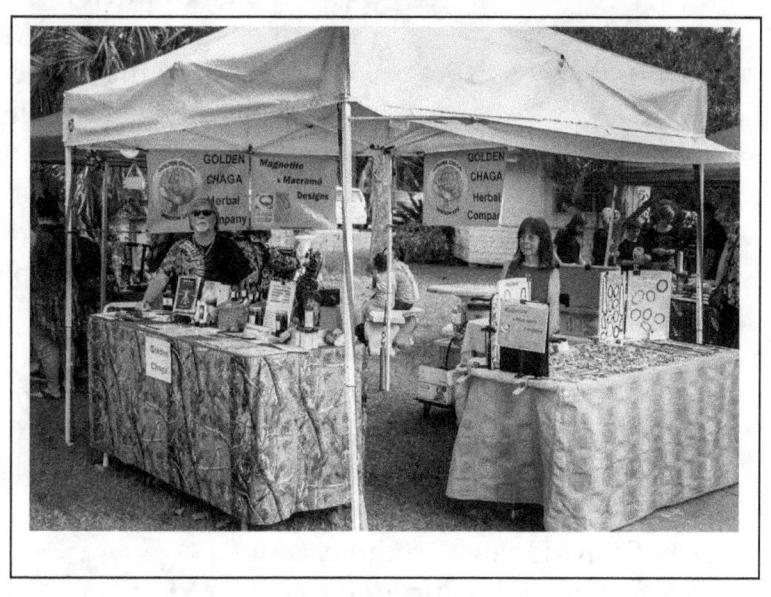

Bon appetite world and best wishes for a vibrant and healthy life!

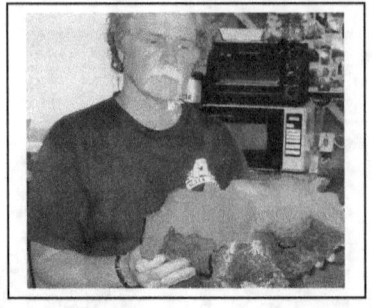

Barry Glidden is a native of the great state of Maine. His life has been an interesting one of diverse occupations and travels - some of which are documented in this book. He and wife, Terry, now live in central Florida in a unique dome habitat - completely off the grid. When first built in 1986 several local television stations aired specials featuring their distinctive style of living. He now focuses his time and talents on harvesting, processing, and marketing Chaga and more importantly, educating people about its benefits.

www.ChagaGoldenProducts.com
info@chagagoldenproducts.com

Margaret Rose Scribner, also a native of New England, now lives in DeLand Florida. Her background is equally diverse. She has owned several retail businesses, most recently an art studio and gallery in DeLand. Since "retiring" she has written, co-authored and illustrated several books, among them are: "Escaping a Life of Quiet Desperation" & "Tales of the Old Moose" (both with son Benjamin), a children's picture book: "Hannah's Incredible Cow", plus "A Sitting Ovation" - an anthology gleaned from a lifetime of her writings - all available on Amazon.

www.scribnerbooksandmore.com

www.ingramcontent.com/pod-product-compliance
Lightning Source LLC
Chambersburg PA
CBHW070106290526
45789CB00005B/1949